About The Author

Gary Stempien has been strength training for 54 years. He is a veteran of the health club industry with a career spanning the last 40 years. Since 1974, he has owned and operated a successful chain of health clubs in the Detroit Metropolitan area, which served thousands of members, including professional athletes from the Detroit Pistons, Detroit Lions, and Detroit Red Wings.

Gary holds a 5th degree black belt in Japanese Ju-Jitsu and Korean Karate, a 1st degree black belt in Kobudo (stick fighting) and Aido (art of the sword), as well as a high ranking brown belt in Aikido. Gary also fought on the Michigan Pro Team for karate and trained in a local boxing club for one year.

Awards Received:

1971 Chung Do Kwan Grand Champion (Sparring) – Mid West Champion

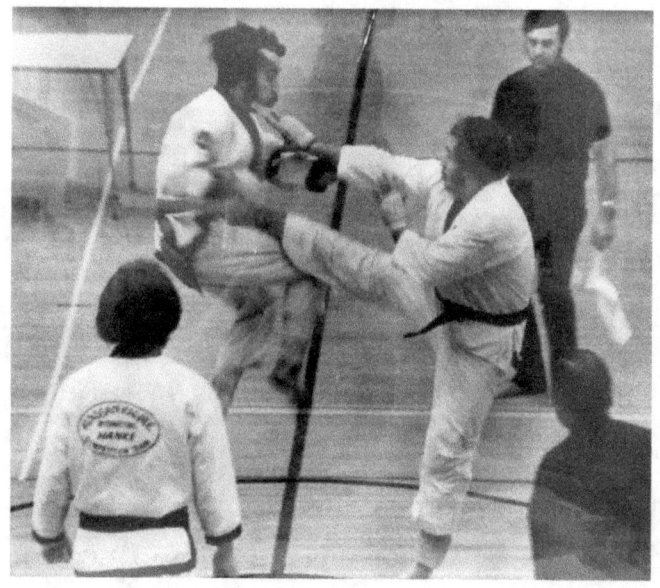

Gary Stempien (right) performing a side kick during a karate competition.

Gary also fought many of the top black belts in the country, including world champion "Super Foot" Bill Wallace. Gary has trained and promoted many students to black belt status, including several masters.

Gary was also a high school football star fullback, receiving all-league and area recognition. Gary had a football scholarship playing for two colleges, two semi-pro teams, and also had a free-agent tryout with the Chicago Bears pro football team.

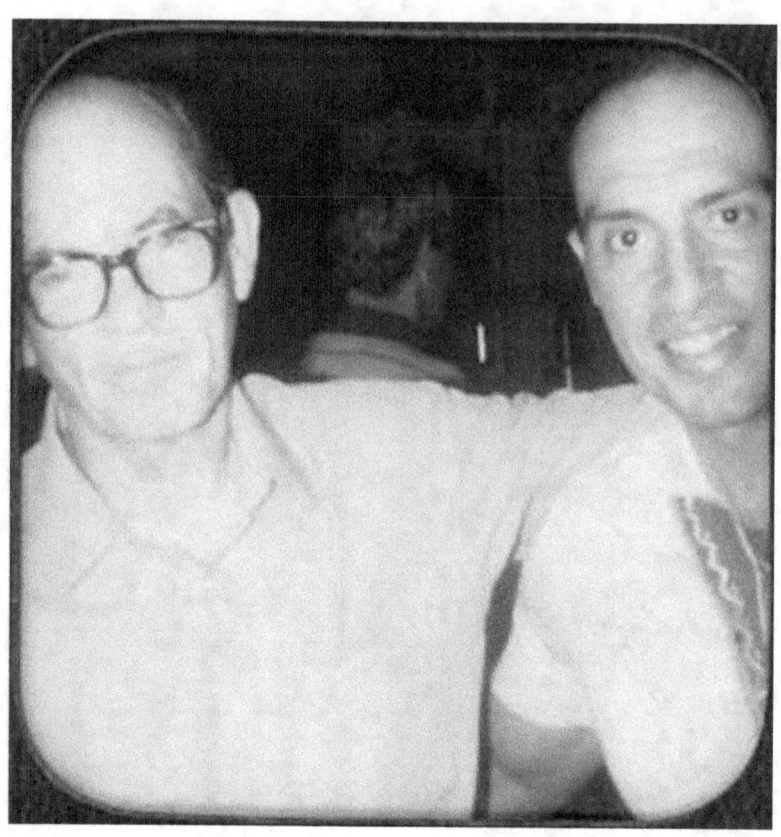

Gary Stempien (right) with his mentor
Arthur Jones (left)

This book is dedicated to my wife, Mary Ann Stempien. We were married two years after I started my business. From the first day we were married, to the present, she has been my guiding light in helping me achieve all of my endeavors. She has been my motivating force.

Introduction

Time is a Factor in Life and Exercise.

55 years ago I started my first type of resistance based exercise. My uncle had given me a Charles Atlas course called "Dynamic Tension". It involved resistance training against your own body parts. As a very young man at the time, I liked how it felt and how my body started to look after following the system.

In 1960, my dad bought me my first set of barbells, and that did it, I started playing the "Iron Game" and I was hooked. My parent's basement became my fulltime gym and I did all that I could to increase my strength and size. I built custom training equipment out of wood, and because steady training partners were hard to come by I made sure to have more than one at all times so there would never be a delay in my training regimen. I consumed all of the information I could find in books and bodybuilding magazines while steadily increasing my techniques and skills to improve my physique.

By the time I was a junior in high school I could bench press 320 pounds and squat 500 pounds. I was easily the strongest guy on the football team, due to the fact that back then very few athletes' strength trained seriously. There was this idea among coaches that strength training would slow and muscle bound. Though this was a very large mistake on their part, it definitely worked to my advantage as one of the few people who realized the many benefits that could be attained from serious, consistent, strength training. It elevated my functional ability in sports to a new level and I reaped the benefits.

Introduction to My Fitness Career

In 1972, I met my mentor, Arthur Jones, the inventor of the Nautilus Fitness Equipment. I spent a large amount of time with Arthur, learning a radical new protocol in strength training that was as ground breaking as it was controversial. As the godfather of modern day strength training equipment, Arthur left a lasting influence on the fitness industry that should not be ignored. Unfortunately, there are few people today in the health club industry who even know who he is.

During my many years in the health club industry I have visited gyms all over the country. In this time I have noticed one recurring theme; the vast majority of people who work out in health clubs have a lacking knowledge of proper strength training, often times leading to many wasted hours that show little to no results. A small percentage of members will hire personal trainers, which is great, but the vast majority of health club members find themselves wandering aimlessly around the machines and weights with no real system or goal to guide them. They have the want and the drive, but what they lack is the time. The time to research training methods, the time to put these methods into practice to find out if they actually work, the time to figure out what their desired level of fitness should be, and even the time to just get into the gym. People who are in good shape and train regularly refer to it as a "lifestyle". Typically, this is because in order to get any worthwhile results out of your workouts your entire life has to revolve around the study and practice that leads to those techniques and skills that produce the best results for you, but is this how it HAS to be? Do you HAVE to be die-hard and live a new "lifestyle" to get results from your training? Why is it that the casual observer, a business professional, working mother, or anyone else with limited available time can't step into a gym and produce decent, worthwhile results in a reasonable amount of time without all of the extra work, study, and uncertainty? I have spent the length of my career trying to find an answer for these questions, and have found a solution in the form of a specialized training system I call the GS20 Express Workout.

The GS20 Express Workout has up to 130 different workouts, designed for anyone from beginners to world-class athletes. Through many years of research and development, tracking thousands of workouts, I have been able to produce consistent and repeatable results. It works, and it works very well. While using the GS20, I have found that the average person has the ability to double their strength in six months.

The workouts are brief, but intense, lasting no longer than 20 minutes when performed correctly. Research shows that it is not the length or duration of the workout that produces the best results, but the intensity or the work performed. So you can train long; up to 1 ½ hours a day, six days a week, or you can train briefly; two to three days a week for 20-30 minutes while producing the same results. The choice is yours.

Are you ready for the challenge? Are you ready to get the body you've always wanted? With the GS20 Express Workout you will get the best results in the least amount of time, safely. This book will guide you through the process, step by step. **Let's get started!**

Your Workout

It is very important to follow specific routines each and every time you work out. Recording everything from weights and repetitions to the date will ensure you achieve great repeatability and consistency in your results. It is the only accurate way to track your gains and make an assessment of your progress. This means no wasted time and effort, just pure results. Recording your progress is also a great way to keep yourself motivated and make every workout more meaningful and challenging.

Research shows that our bodies respond best to a variety of exercises and challenges. As far as the GS20 is concerned, variety can be defined as performing a different routine every time you work out. Challenges can be defined as implementing "progressive overload". When you increase your weights so that your muscles consistently experience this overload the body has to defend itself and it does so through hypertrophy, that is becoming stronger and more efficient. In other words: more muscle, less fat, greater heart-lung capacity, and increased base metabolic rate. The body becomes a charged up fat burner.

So how many repetitions should you be performing to overload your muscles? A rep should take roughly seven seconds to complete. Two seconds on the lifting phase (positive motion) and four seconds on the return phase (negative motion). Therefore ten reps would take 70 seconds, and your time under workload should be within 84 seconds, which equates to twelve reps. This "rep range" gives you the best anabolic training effect. Train any more than that and you will reach your aerobic threshold.

A Basic Explanation

There will be 4 different workouts: Beginner, Intermediate, Advanced, and a modified shorter workout called the "Max Body Blast". There is only a small window of opportunity when the body actually builds muscle, anything more than that and you are expending a lot of needless energy. Even worse, when you over train you are creating a deep inroad into your recovery ability. Inroad is the momentary loss of strength from a set of exercises. Therefore the body will produce higher levels of cortisol, which is a stress hormone brought on by mental and physical stress. This in turn throws your body into a deep catabolic state. In this state you will never build muscle, in fact, you will end up losing muscle!

The GS20 is designed to keep you from over-training and therefore keeps your body from entering that catabolic state. When in a catabolic state your body is exhausted, which in turn affects your drive and energy to consistently workout and produce results. By keeping your body in an efficient anabolic state you will consistently produce results and keep yourself on track.

It cannot be stressed enough that the need to record your workouts, repetitions, and other details like seat settings and workout times is absolutely crucial to your success with this program. This will establish consistency in your training, thereby making your workouts more meaningful and challenging.

Time to Work Out!

I will repeat myself throughout this book on a few key points in order to drive home just how important they are. Each repetition must be performed slowly; two seconds on the lifting phase (positive) and four second on the lowering phase (negative). Hold for one second at the end of the lifting phase on all exercises, with the exception of pressing movements (leg press, chest press, overhead press, etc). Pressing movements should be performed non-stop with no pause at the end of the lifting phase. This keeps the workload constant on the targeted muscle groups.

Selectorized Weight Machine Workouts

Beginner Workout

1st Workout:

Leg Curl

Leg Extension

Leg Press (or Squat)

Pullover

Lat Pull Down

Chest press

Bicep

Tricep

Abdominal Machine

Muscle Building and Fat Cutting: 10-minute interval on cardio machine ("Hard Gainers" (Individuals that have trouble gaining weight) avoid cardio)

2nd Workout:

Leg Extension

Leg Curl

Inner Thigh (Adduction)

Outer Thigh (Abduction)

Lat. Pull Down

Lateral Raise

Pec Fly

Abdominal Machine

Tricep

Bicep

Muscle Building and Fat Cutting: 10-minute interval on cardio machine (Hard Gainers avoid cardio)

3rd Workout:

Inner Thigh (Adduction)

Leg Extension

Leg Press (or Squat)

Pullover

Lat Pull Down

Lateral Raise

Pec Fly

Tricep

Bicep

Abdominal Machine

Muscle Building and Fat Cutting: 10-minute interval on cardio machine (Hard Gainers avoid cardio)

Intermediate Workout

1st Workout:

Leg Curl

Leg Extension

Leg Press (or Squat)

Outer Thigh (Abduction)

Pullover

Lat Pull Down

Overhead Press

Chest Press

Bicep

Assisted Dips (Gravitron Machine)

Abdominal Machine

Hip Flexion (Slowly lift your knees to your chest on the hip flexion bar. If one is not available grab the cross bar of a chin up bar at arms length, then slowly lift your knees to your chest.

Neck Machine (if available)

Muscle Building and Fat Cutting: 10-minute interval on cardio machine (Hard Gainers avoid cardio)

2nd Workout:

Leg Extension

Leg Curl

Inner Thigh (Adduction)

Outer Thigh (Abduction)

Low Row

Lateral Raise

Pec Fly

Abdominal Machine

Tricep

Wrist Curls (With Dumbbells)

Calf-Raise

No Cardio

3<u>rd</u> <u>Workout:</u>

Inner Thigh (Adduction)

Leg Press (or Squat)

Leg Extension

Leg Press (or Squat)

Pullover

Low Row

Lateral Raise

Pec Fly

Tricep

Bicep

Assisted Chins (Gravitron Machine)

Abdominal Machine

Muscle Building and Fat Cutting: 10-minute interval on cardio machine (Hard Gainers avoid cardio)

Note: At the intermediate and advanced level you should start including "post-fatigue" reps at the end of each exercise. To perform a post-fatigue rep you immediately lower the weight of the exercise you just finished (20lbs on upper body exercises and 40lbs on lower body exercises) and perform an additional 2-4 repetitions. This will activate a reserve of slow twitch muscle fibers, thereby stimulating all of your available muscle fibers.

Advanced Workout

<u>1st workout:</u>

Leg Curl

Leg Ext

Leg Press (or Squat)

Outer Thigh (Abduction)

Pullover

Lat Pull Down

Overhead Press

Chest Press

Bicep

Assisted Dips (Gravitron Machine)

Abdominal Machine

Hip Flexion (Slowly lift your knees to your chest on the hip

flexion bar. If one is not available grab the cross bar of a chin up bar at arm's length, then slowly lift your knees to your chest.

Neck Machine (if available)

Muscle Building and Fat Cutting: 10-minute interval on cardio machine (Hard Gainers avoid cardio)

As noted on intermediate level, perform post fatigue reps on all exercises.

2nd <u>workout</u>:

Leg Extensions

Leg Curl

Inner Thigh (Adduction)

Outer Thigh (Abduction)

Lat Pull Down

Lateral Raise

Pec Fly

Abdominal Machine

Tricep

Wrist Curls

Calf Raise

Muscle Building and Fat Cutting: 10-minute interval on cardio machine (Hard Gainers avoid cardio)

3rd workout:

Inner Thigh (Adduction)

Leg Press (or Squat)

Leg Extensions

Leg Press (or Squat. Perform this exercise at a lower weight than the previous one)

Lat Pull Down

Lateral Raise

Pec Fly

Tricep

Bicep

Dips (Negative Only)

Negatives Explanation: Negative training is training that focuses on the negative (or return) portion of an exercise. This can be a tricky exercise to pull off if you do not have the proper equipment, but here is how you can use it while you perform dips. First you will need a weight belt with a chain, and a gravitron machine or a simple dip bar with a step stool. Begin by placing your hands on the dip bars. Place the knee platform at very bottom of machine (if using gravitron machine). Secure your weight discs through chain, walk up the stairs – arms locked out – then begin bending your arms and slowly lower your body. Try to go as low as you can for a count of eight full seconds – now walk back up the stairs and immediately start rep two. Perform 8-12 repetitions

Note: The lifting phase (positive) is performed by walking back up the stairs. All of your strength should be used on the negative phase of the exercise.

Negative Chins: Also use a gravitron machine or a chin up bar with a stool. Place your hands on the chinning bar, using the weight belt as you did with the negative dips. Now walk up the stairs and lower your body until your arms are fully extended for a count of eight seconds, till your arms are fully extended. Walk back up the stairs and immediately start rep two. Continue for 8-12 reps.

Assisted chins: Again use a gravitron machine. Lift your body for a count of two seconds then lower your body for a count of four seconds. Perform 8-12 reps. Because you are using a gravitron machine you can choose the amount of weight you want to assist you with the exercise. With this machine though you want to be sure to lower the weight as you get stronger so that eventually you are lifting and lowering your fully body weight.

Max Body Blast!

Leg Extension

Leg Press

Pullover

Lat Pull Down

Bicep

Negative Dips

Note: Be sure to move immediately from leg extension to leg press with no rest between the two exercises. Once completed, get a drink of water or just rest for 30 seconds before moving on. Move immediately from pullover to lat pull down, and don't forget the post fatigue reps!

Selectorized to Free-Weight Training

I prefer selectorized weight machines to free-weights because there is a significant difference in the time and safety factors. These workouts are maximum intensity workouts, so on some free weight exercises you would need a spotter. As I learned when I was younger, having someone to work out with all the time is not reliable, and not everyone can keep multiple training partners on call at all times. Even if you did always have a training partner the time spent switching out weights extends the workout period significantly. I have found that results comparing the machines to the free weights are the same, so the preference on which to use is really up to you.

I will include free weight routines for those wanting them. These routines are one set workouts. Through the years I have tried different training protocols, both on myself and with many other subjects. These studies, and the results produced, have convinced me that the single set, high intensity, protocol is the preferred one. Research shows that when you take a set to failure you have involved all of the available muscle fibers, when you rest and perform another set you have just reactivated the same muscle fibers. The more sets you perform the deeper of an inroad you create into your recovery ability. Therefore it will take you much longer to recover from that workout.

With single set training, you will stimulate the maximum amount of muscle fibers, recover much quicker between workouts, and stimulate much more muscle growth. When using the GS20 program, you should rest at least 48 hours minimum between each workout and a maximum of 96 hours. The stronger you get the more time you need to take to fully recover from your workouts in order to make maximum gains.

My very advanced trainees' workout only twice a week, performing only the 1st and 3rd workouts and utilizing the maximum 96 hours of recovery time. This is because their workouts are so intense that they need the extra recovery time between workouts to maintain their effectiveness. In my earlier years I over trained for quite a long time. I finally came to the conclusion that I had wasted a lot of time and energy and produced few results. The GS20 method will allow you to produce maximal results in the minimum time required.

GS20 Free Weight Workout

These workouts are for those who may not have access to all of the machines mentioned in previous workouts, or for those who prefer using free-weights as well as machines. Where no suitable free-weight exercise is available a machine is listed as its replacement to ensure you still get a full body workout. Most gyms have these machines available as they are considered staples in the health club industry.

Beginner
Workout

1st Workout:

Leg Curl (Machine)

Leg Extension (Machine)

Barbell Squat or Hip Sled

Bent-Over Row (Barbell)

Lat Pull Down (Machine)

Overhead Press -Seated barbell or dumbbell, or plate

loaded machine if available

Bench Press

Bicep – Standing barbell curl or preacher curl

Tricep – Tricep push downs, lat machine, or close hand

bench press

Abdominal (Machine)

Muscle Building and Fat Cutting: 10-minute interval on cardio machine (Hard Gainers avoid cardio)

2nd Workout:

Leg Extension (Machine)

Leg Curl (Machine)

Inner Thigh (Machine)

Outer Thigh (Machine)

Low Row (Machine)

Lateral Raise -Standing lateral dumbbell raise

Pec Fly – Flat bench dumbbell flys

Abdominal (Machine)

Tricep – Tricep push downs, lat machine, or close hand bench press

Bicep – Standing barbell curl or preacher curl

3rd Workout:

Inner Thigh (Machine)

Leg Extension (Machine)

Hack Squat – Hip Sled

Leg Curl (Machine)

One arm bent over dumbbell row

Low Row (Machine)

Lateral Raise -Standing lateral dumbbell raise

Pec Fly – Cable cross over (Machine)

Tricep – Dips on dip machine or dip bar

Bicep – Standing dumbbell curls

Abdominal (Machine)

Muscle Building and Fat Cutting: 10-minute interval on cardio machine (Hard Gainers avoid cardio)

Intermediate Workout

1st Workout:

Leg Curl (Machine)

Leg Extension (Machine)

Leg Press (Machine)

Outer Thigh (Machine)

Bent-Over Row (Barbell)

Low Row (Machine)

Overhead Press -Seated barbell or dumbbell, or plate loaded machine if available

Bench Press

Bicep – Standing barbell curl or preacher curl

Dips – Dip machine or dip bar

Abdominal (Machine)

Hip Flexion (Slowly lift your knees to your chest on the hip flexion bar. If one is not available grab the cross bar of a chin up bar at arm's length, then slowly lift your knees to your chest.)

Neck machine (if available)

2nd Workout:

Leg Extension (Machine)

Leg Curl (Machine)

Inner Thigh (Machine)

Outer Thigh (Machine)

Lat Pull High Row

Pec Fly – Flat bench dumbbell flys

Abdominal (Machine)

Tricep – Tricep push downs, lat machine, or close hand bench press

Wrist Curls – Dumbbell

Calf Raise – Seated calf machine

3rd Workout:

Inner Thigh (Machine)

Leg Press – Hip Sled

Leg Extension (Machine)

Barbell squat

Barbell bent-over row

Lat Pull Down (Machine)

Lateral Raise -Standing lateral dumbbell raise

Pec Fly – Flat bench flys

Tricep – Dips on dip machine or dip bar

Bicep – Concentrating curls, one arm

Abdominal – Floor crunches

Muscle Building and Fat Cutting: 10-minute interval on cardio machine (Hard Gainers avoid cardio)

Advanced Workout

1st Workout:

Leg Curl (Machine)

Leg Extension (Machine)

Hack Squat – Hip sled

Outer Thigh (Machine)

Chin ups on chinning bar

High Row – Lat machine

Overhead Press -Seated barbell or dumbbell, or plate loaded machine if available

Bench Press

Bicep – Standing, alternating, bicep curls

Assisted Dips – Gravitron machine

Abdominal (Machine)

Neck Machine (If available)

2nd Workout:

Leg Extensions (Machine)

Leg Curl (Machine)

Inner Thigh (Machine)

Outer Thigh (Machine)

Lat Pull Down (Machine)

Lateral Raise – Seated dumbbell raises

Pec Fly – Flat bench flys

Abdominal – Floor crunches

Wrist Curls – Dumbbells

3rd Workout:

Inner Thigh (Machine)

Hack Squat – Hip sled

Leg Extensions (Machine)

Barbell squat

Chin ups on chinning bar

Lateral Raise -Standing lateral dumbbell raise

Pec Fly – Flat bench flys

Tricep – Tricep push downs, lat machine, or close hand bench press

Bicep – Preacher curls

Negative Dips (Refer to the selectorized machine workouts, third workout, or advanced section for explanation)

Negative Chins (Refer to the selectorized machine workouts, third workout, or advanced section for explanation)

Assisted Chins – Gravitron machine

Abdominal – Floor crunches

Performing with Intensity

Are you enjoying your workouts? If you are then you're not working hard enough! Perform each rep as if your life depended on it. Have pure concentration with each and every rep you perform. Feel those muscle fibers contracting. It is the last few reps when you really start to challenge your body's pain threshold. It's at that point the targeted muscle will send a neuromuscular response to the brain telling your body to stop what it is doing. The next rep after that is the most important, it's at this moment when you will be stimulating a reserve of muscular fibers and begin triggering muscular growth.

I have observed many subjects throughout the years, and large amounts have never experienced a "maximum intensity workout". That is why many of them end up over training in an attempt to compensate for the lack of intensity in their workouts. They don't put in the necessary work and don't see the results they want, so they over work themselves mistakenly believing it will provide results. You get out what you put in and nothing more.

After a few workouts you can begin to track your progress and see your strength increase. You will begin seeing an increase in muscle mass as your body fat decreases. Just look in the mirror and see for yourself, it doesn't lie, and you will like what you see!

Tracking Your Progress

As I mentioned earlier in this book, in order to truly know if you are making progress in your workouts you must track what you are doing. The process is simple but in order for it to be effective you must keep accurate and consistent records. Once you have performed all of the workouts at least once you can begin challenging yourself by looking at the results from the previous week and attempting to do better. If you performed 10 reps the last time try and get 12 this time, and if you get those 12 reps raise the weight by five pounds for next time. This is how progress is made, and if you are keeping accurate records you can see an immediate increase in your strength and endurance. The ability to see your progress like this is a great motivator and one of the major benefits of accurate record keeping.

Motivation

I grew up in a very modest middle class environment. My dad worked at a cemetery in the 1940's. He had to dig the graves by hand with a shovel, and during the winters he would have to use a jackhammer to break apart the frozen earth. Needless to say my dad worked very hard to support our family.

My parents were very gracious, giving us what they could; we lived from week to week. I quickly realized that life was not going to be easy and they only way to get anywhere was through consistent hard work, a lesson I took to heart when I worked to pay my way through college.

In 1972, a friend and I were living in Florida painting apartments when I heard about Arthur Jones and his bizarre exercise machines. Arthur had, at that time, only a few pieces of equipment out of the prototype phase but they were already making waves in the fitness industry. My friend and I were intrigued so we decide to visit Arthur in DeLand at his manufacturing plant. That visit changed my life forever.

For the next two years I visited Arthur on a regular basis, learning everything I possibly could from him. He was a brilliant man, truly a genius. What Arthur was teaching me was cutting edge, a new training protocol that would change strength training forever.

After several years of study and training, and with Arthur's encouragement, I decided to open my first health club. However, I was still a struggling college student with little to no savings to start any sort of business with. Eventually my grandmother was kind enough to loan me $2000 as a starting investment for my business; my friend, who then became my business partner, also invested an additional $2000. Though it was a start, this small sum was nowhere near enough money to start our business with. Once again, Arthur had the solution. He suggested that I meet a friend of his, a man named P.M. Strickland, who lived in Columbus, Georgia. I was extremely motivated to get this business off the ground so my friend and I jumped into our old rickety painting van and started our trek from the Detroit area to Columbus, Georgia. After we had been driving all day we pulled into a motel parking lot, but we only had enough money for food and fuel, so rather than getting a room we opted to sleep in the van. In the morning we snuck into the motel's pool to rinse off then got back on the road towards Georgia.

Meeting Mr. Strickland was an experience I will never forget. He was a grey bearded man with a thick southern accent who reminded me of Colonel Sanders. Minutes after we had arrived at his office his phone rang. Mr. Strickland answered it and said "Yes Arthur those boys are here!" after which Arthur immediately hung up on him. Mr. Strickland then looked at us and said, "You boys are now young business men!" Mr. Strickland, as it turns out, was a financier who Arthur had convinced to invest in our first health club. He arranged all of the financing for our first line of equipment.

A month after that visit we opened our first gym in Madison Heights, Michigan. Our equipment hadn't arrived yet but we were anxious to begin so we set up various pictures of the equipment we were going to be receiving and began pre-selling memberships based entirely on the premise of the training principals I had learned from Arthur Jones. Shortly afterwards our equipment arrived and we began training people.

I was ready to explode with enthusiasm and a desire to succeed! Never for even a second did I think that I was not going to be successful. Within the next year and a half we opened two more gyms, with many more to follow after. People traveled from all over the area to try my bizarre training system, which were the very beginnings of the GS20 Express Workout. Ultimately, I owe Arthur Jones for my career in this industry.

You can do this! You will do this! With a little self-motivation and a huge amount of effort when performing these very brief workouts you will get results you never thought possible. The hardest part of any endeavor is starting. When it's time to train you've got to buckle down and just begin.

Workouts Week 5-8

Selectorized Weight Machine Workouts

Beginner
Workout

1st Workout:

Leg Curl

Leg Extension

Leg Press (or Squat)

Inner Thigh

Lat. pulldown

Pec Fly

Chest press

Lateral Raise

Overhead press

Abdominal

Tricep

Bicep

Muscle Building and Fat Cutting: 10-minute interval on cardio machine (Hard Gainers avoid cardio)

2nd Workout:

Leg Curl

Leg Press (or Squat)

Inner Thigh

Outer Thigh

Lat. Pulldown

Lateral Raise

Pec Fly

Overhead Press

Abdominal

Bicep

Tricep

Muscle Building and Fat Cutting: 10-minute interval on cardio machine (Hard Gainers avoid cardio)

<u>3rd Workout:</u>

Leg Curl

Leg Press (or Squat)

Leg Extension

Outer Thigh

Lat. Pulldown

Pullover (or Low Row)

Chest Press

Overhead Press

Bicep

Tricep

Abdominal

Muscle Building and Fat Cutting: 10-minute interval on cardio machine (Hard Gainers avoid cardio)

Intermediate
Workout

1st Workout:

Leg Curl

Leg Extension

Leg Press

Inner Thigh

Low Row

Pec Fly

Chest Press

Lateral Raise

Overhead Press

Abdominal

Tricep

Assisted Chins (Gravitron)

Muscle Building and Fat Cutting: 10-minute interval on cardio machine (Hard Gainers avoid cardio)

2nd Workout:

Leg Curl

Leg Press (or Squat)

Inner Thigh

Outer Thigh

Lat. Pulldown

Pec Fly

Overhead Press

Abdominal

Bicep

Calf-Raise (seated calf-raise machine)

Wrist-Curls (with dumbbell)

Neck machine (if available)

Muscle Building and Fat Cutting: 10-minute interval on cardio machine (Hard Gainers avoid cardio)

3rd Workout:

Leg Curl

Leg Press (NA) Note: Negative Accentuated – Lift with two legs (positive) lower with one leg (negative) for a count of eight seconds. Perform the same motion for the second rep, only this time lower the weight with the opposite leg as before. Perform four to six repetitions with each leg.

Leg Extension

Leg Press (or Squat)

Outer Thigh

Lat. Pulldown

Pullover (or Low Row)

Chest Press

Overhead Press

Bicep

Assisted Dips (Gravitron)

Abdominal

Muscle Building and Fat Cutting: 10-minute interval on cardio machine (Hard Gainers avoid cardio)

Advanced Workout

1st Workout:

Leg Curl

Leg Extension

Leg Press

Inner Thigh

Pullover (or Low Row)

Lat. Pull Down

Chest Press

Lateral Raise

Incline Press

Abdominal

Tricep

Assisted Chins

Muscle Building and Fat Cutting: 10-minute interval on cardio machine (Hard Gainers avoid cardio)

2nd Workout:

Leg Curl

Leg Press (or Squat)

Inner Thigh

Outer Thigh

Lat. Pulldown

Pec Fly

Incline Press

Abdominal

Bicep

Calf-Raise (seated calf-raise machine)

Wrist-Curls (with dumbbell) Note: Place your entire forearm on your lap, movement should come just from your wrists.

Neck machine (if available)

Muscle Building and Fat Cutting: 10-minute interval on cardio machine (Hard Gainers avoid cardio)

3rd Workout:

Buns of Steel Workout!

Leg Curl

Leg press (NA) Note: Negative Accentuated – Lift with two legs (positive) lower with one leg (negative) for a count of eight seconds. Perform the same motion for the second rep, only this time lower the weight with the opposite leg as before. Perform four to six repetitions with each leg.

Leg Extension (Super Slow) Lift with both legs for a count of ten seconds, lower both legs for a count of four seconds. Perform no more than 4-6 reps!

Leg Press (Normal)

Outer Thigh

Lat. Pulldown

Negative Chins: Also use a gravitron machine or a chin up bar with a stool. Place your hands on the chinning bar, using the weight belt as you did with the negative dips. Now walk up the stairs and lower your body until your arms are fully extended for a count of 8 seconds, till your arms are fully extended. Walk back up the stairs and immediately start rep 2. Continue for 8-12 reps.

Pec Fly

Negative Dips: Begin by placing your hands on the dip bars.

Place the knee platform at very bottom of machine (if using gravitron machine). Secure your weight discs through chain, walk up the stairs – arms locked out – then begin bending your arms and slowly lower your body. Try to go as low as you can for a count of eight full seconds – now walk back up the stairs and immediately start rep two. Perform 8-12 repetitions

Lateral Raise

Bicep

Assisted Dips (Gravitron)

Muscle Building and Fat Cutting: 10-minute interval on cardio machine (Hard Gainers avoid cardio)

Max Body Blast!

Note: Remember to occasionally perform one of these workouts instead of the 3rd workout in order to shock your muscles!

Leg Press

Leg Extension

Lat Pull Down

Assisted Chins

Overhead Press

Assisted Dips

Note: Be sure to move immediately from leg extension to leg press with no rest between the two exercises. Once completed, get a drink of water or just rest for 30 seconds before moving on. Move immediately from pullover to lat pull down, and don't forget the post fatigue reps!

GS20 Free Weight Routines

Beginner Workout

1st Workout:

Leg Curl (Machine)

Leg Extension (Machine)

Hack Squat (Machine)

Inner Thigh (Machine)

Flat Bench Dumbbell Flys

Bench Press

Standing Lateral Dumbbell Raises

Incline Dumbbell Presses (Incline Bench)

Abdominal (Floor Crunches)

Close Hand Bench Press – Note: keep hands 6" apart

Standing Alternate Dumbbell Curls

Muscle Building and Fat Cutting: 10-minute interval on cardio machine (Hard Gainers avoid cardio)

2nd Workout:

Leg Curl (Machine)

Leg Press (Hip Sled)

Inner Thigh (Machine)

Outer Thigh (Machine)

One Arm Bent Over Row with Dumbbell

Seated Lateral Raise with Dumbbells

Standing Cable Flys (Cable Cross-Over Machine)

Seated Overhead Press (Flat Bench)

Abdominal (Machine)

Preacher Curls

Tricep Kick Backs - Dumbbells

Muscle Building and Fat Cutting: 10-minute interval on cardio machine (Hard Gainers avoid cardio)

3rd Workout:

Leg Curl (Machine)

Barbell Squats (use power rack or smith machine)

Leg Extension (Machine)

Outer Thigh (Machine)

Lat. Pull Down (Machine)

Bent Over Row (Barbell)

Bench Press

Incline Press with Dumbbells (Incline Bench)

Bicep – seated one-arm concentration dumbbell curls

Tricep – dips on dip bar

Abdominal (Machine)

Muscle Building and Fat Cutting: 10-minute interval on cardio machine (Hard Gainers avoid cardio)

Intermediate
Workout

<u>1st Workout:</u>

Leg Curl (Machine)

Leg Extension (Machine)

Barbell Squat (power rack or smith machine)

Inner Thigh (Machine)

Lat. Pull Down (Machine)

Pec fly (Dumbbell Flys on Flat Bench)

Bench Press

Seated Lateral Dumbbell Raises

Incline Dumbbell Press (Incline Bench)

Abdominal (Machine)

Tricep Push Downs (Lat. Machine)

Assisted Chins (Gravitron)

Muscle Building and Fat Cutting: 10-minute interval on cardio machine (Hard Gainers avoid cardio)

2nd Workout:

Leg Curl (Machine)

Hack Squat (Machine, plate loaded)

Inner Thigh (Machine)

Outer Thigh (Machine)

One Arm Bent Over Row with Dumbbell

Pec Fly (Machine)

Seated Dumbbell Incline Press (Incline Bench)

Floor Crunches

Bicep   standing barbell curls

Calf-Raise (seated calf machine)

Seated Barbell Wrist Curls

Neck – Neck Machine, if available

Muscle Building and Fat Cutting: 10-minute interval on cardio machine (Hard Gainers avoid cardio)

3rd Workout:

Leg Curl (Machine)

Hip Sled Leg Press (NA) - refer to 3rd workout selectorized machine workout for negative accentuated details

Leg Extensions (Super Slow) – refer to intermediate workout #3 selectorized machine workout

Barbell Squat (power rack or smith machine)

Lat. Pull Down

Bent Over Barbell Row

Bench Press

Incline Barbell Press (Incline Bench)

Bicep (Preacher Curl Bench)

Assisted Dips (Gravitron)

Muscle Building and Fat Cutting: 10-minute interval on cardio machine (Hard Gainers avoid cardio)

Advanced Workout

1st Workout:

Leg Curl (Machine)

Leg Extension (Machine)

Hack Squat (Hip Sled Machine)

Inner Thigh (Machine)

Barbell Bent Over Row (palm up)

Lat. Pull Down (Machine)

Bench Press

Lateral Dumbbell Raise (seated)

Seated Overhead Press – barbell

Floor Crunches

Tricep Push Downs (Lat. Machine)

Assisted Chins (Gravitron)

Muscle Building and Fat Cutting: 10-minute interval on cardio machine (Hard Gainers avoid cardio)

2nd Workout:

Leg Curl (Machine)

Barbell Squat (power rack or smith machine)

Inner Thigh (Machine)

Outer Thigh (Machine)

One Arm Bent Over Row with Dumbbell

Pec Fly (cable cross over)

Overhead Press (seated dumbbells)

Floor Crunches

Bicep – standing barbell curls

Calf Raises (seated calf machine)

Wrist Curls – seated barbell wrist curls

Neck (Machine, if available)

Muscle Building and Fat Cutting: 10-minute interval on cardio machine (Hard Gainers avoid cardio)

3rd Workout:

Leg Curl (Machine)

Leg Press (NA, Hip Sled) – refer to selectorized 3rd workout – intermediate

Leg Extension (Super Slow) – refer to selectorized 3rd workout – intermediate

Barbell Squat (power rack or smith machine)

Outer Thigh (Machine)

Lat. Pull Down (Lat. Machine)

Negative Chins – refer to 3rd workout selectorized machines, advanced

Pec Fly – dumbbell flys, flat bench

Negative Dips - refer to 3rd workout selectorized

machines, advanced

Lateral Raise – seated dumbbells

Bicep – preacher curl

Assisted Dips (Gravitron)

Muscle Building and Fat Cutting: 10-minute interval on cardio

machine (Hard Gainers avoid cardio)

Max Body Blast!

Note: Remember to occasionally perform one of these workouts instead of the 3rd workout in order to shock your muscles!

Leg Extension (Machine)

Note: Have the first two exercises pre-set in order to move more quickly from exercises to exercise.

Leg Press (Hip Sled)

Lat. Pull down (Machine)

Barbell Bent Over Row

Bicep (Preacher Curl)

Assisted Dips (Gravitron)

Note: Be sure to move immediately from leg extension to leg press with no rest between the two exercises. Once completed, get a drink of water or just rest for 30 seconds before moving on. Move immediately from pullover to lat pull down, and don't forget the post fatigue reps!

Glossary

GS20 Max Body blast – Abbreviated workout consisting of six exercises.

Catabolic – Breakdown state.

Anabolic – Building state.

Inroad – Momentary loss of strength from a set of an exercise.

Cortisol – A stress hormone, brought on by mental and physical stress.

Metabolic Equilibrium – Blood sugar at its most efficient level, when eating a meal every three hours.

Positive – The lifting phase when performing an exercise.

Negative – The lowering phase when performing an exercise.

Fiber Recruitment Pattern – The order and type of muscle fibers that contract from the start of an exercise to the end of an exercise.

Volitional Fatigue – Also known as "Momentary Muscular Failure". When performing an exercise and your level of strength drops below the level of resistance.

Super Slow – Lifting a weight for a count of ten seconds, then lowering the weight for a count of four seconds, performing 4-6 repetitions.

Negative Accentuated – Lifting with two limbs, then lowering with one limb, alternating on each repetition. Perform 4-6 reps on each side. Lifting phase should take two seconds, lowering phase should take eight seconds.

Negative only – Lower the weight for a count of eight seconds, perform 8-12 repetitions.

Pre Exhaustion Principle – Moving immediately from a single joint movement to a multiple joint movement. Example: Leg extension to leg press, pullover to lat. pull down, pec fly to chest press, lateral raise to overhead press.

Appendix

Nutrition and Your Workout

To achieve the best possible results in your workouts your nutrition is vitally important. In fact, your nutrition is 100% equally important as your workouts!

Through the years I have discussed nutrition with literally thousands of my members, and in most cases I reach the same conclusion: They really do not concentrate on their nutrition. This truly does have a direct impact on the level of results that they will achieve in their workouts. Think about it, you have to eat to live, so with a little bit of planning you can develop a nutrition plan for a lifetime. Yes, a lifestyle change that also includes a cutting edge strength training system that is quick, efficient, and safe.

It is very important to eat six meals a day approximately every three hours. By doing so you will maintain metabolic equilibrium, the body's most efficient blood-sugar level. In this state you will lose fat and build muscle, keeping your body anabolic (build up state).

To establish metabolic equilibrium you must have a complete meal consisting of protein, fats, and carbohydrates. For example, a sandwich with multi-grain bread, turkey, a slice of Swiss-cheese, a spread, a glass of low-fat milk and a piece of fruit.

Supplements

Supplementation will take your training to a new level as well as helping to make meal planning easy.

In the last 15 years the development of nutritional supplements has greatly improved, producing some really good companies with high quality products. I take a pre-workout drink about 40 minutes before my workout, an intra drink during my workout, and a post-workout drink immediately after my workout. This combination allows me to get the most out of my workouts, and they do work. I track all of my workouts and because of this I can tell that every time I train with supplements I manage to get plus reps. This leads me to believe that the effects of these supplements are truly physiological, not just psychological.

Multi Vitamins and Minerals

Our foods today are not the same as they were a half a century ago. They have been abused by the big agricultural companies by over cultivation, the over use of pesticides, and overuse of chemical fertilizers. Our produce has been genetically modified, plus increased time and distance from the farm to the table decreases the amount of nutrients available in our foods. These problems therefore make it necessary to take a high quality multi vitamin and mineral supplement daily.

When choosing a multi vitamin and mineral supplement, it is best to use only products that list actual foods as their ingredients rather than synthetic and isolated vitamins, such as acerola cherry powder instead of vitamin c.

Macronutrients

Protein – Proteins are actually made up of amino acids, which are the building blocks of our body tissue.

There are 20 different types of amino acids and they are divided into three different groups; essential amino acids, non-essential amino acids, and conditional amino acids.

Essential amino acids cannot be made by the body, therefore it is essential to have them in our diet. Non-essential amino acids are made by the body from essential amino acids. Conditional amino acids are only needed during times of illness or stress.

Protein sources are grouped according to how many essential amino acids they contain. Complete proteins contain all of the essential amino acids. Animal based foods like beef, chicken, fish, eggs, milk and cheese would be considered complete proteins. Incomplete protein sources lack one or more of the essential amino acids.

Carbohydrates – The main role of carbohydrates is to provide energy to the cells of the body. There are three forms of carbohydrates: Simple carbs (sugars), complex carbs (starches), and fiber.

Simple carbs are found in sugary foods like fruit, milk, and vegetables. They are also found in refined and processed foods such as candy, soda, and table sugar. Refined sugars provide calories but lack vitamins, minerals, and fiber. Often referred to as "empty calories" and can lead to weight gain.

Complex carbs include starchy vegetables, legumes, and whole gain breads and cereals. Fibrous carbs come from vegetables and fruit. These foods are low glycemic, which enter the blood stream more slowly. Eating fat or protein with the carbohydrates will also slow digestion and decrease the glycemic content of the food.

Processed carbs, refined foods, and added sugars are more likely to raise your sugar level quickly (high glycemic).

Fats - Fats are a source of fuel energy and helps the body absorb fat-soluble vitamins. Fats are made up of three groups: mono-unsaturated fat, poly-unsaturated fat, and trans fat.

Mono-unsaturated fats have one double-carbon bond, as opposed to poly-unsaturated fats that have multiple double bonds. These fats can reduce "bad" cholesterol in your blood. Mono-unsaturated fat is helpful for weight loss because it promotes the feeling of fullness making it easier to adhere to your diet plan.

Poly-unsaturated fats have multiple double bonds. Both poly-unsaturated and mono-unsaturated fats are believed to lower cholesterol. Good sources include corn oil, soybean oil, fatty fish like salmon and tuna, seeds like sunflower and pumpkin.

Saturated fats can come from things like high fat meats like beef, pork, and chicken, lard, whole fat milk, cream, butter and cheese.

Trans-fats include hydrogenated fats which are a part of many processed foods such as commercially made snacks like cookies, doughnuts, crackers, chips, and candy bars. They are also found in commercially fried foods such as fried chicken, chicken nuggets, french fries, and hydrogenated fats like margarine, turning a good food into a bad food.

Fat is essential to our diet. Vitamins A, D, E, and K are fat soluble, meaning that they can only be digested, absorbed, and transported in conjunction with fats. Fats are also sources of essential fatty acids, which are important dieting requirements.

Omega 3 and 6 are essential fatty acids, or EFA's, that humans and other animals must eat because the body requires them for good health and our bodies cannot manufacture them. Olive oil is rich in omega 6, and fish oil is also high in omega 3.

Fiber- Fiber refers to carbohydrates that that cannot be digested. Fiber is present in all plants that are eaten for food such as fruits, vegetables, grains, and legumes. Fiber is an important part of a healthy diet.

Both soluble and insoluble fibers are essential to any diet. Examples of soluble fiber include oatmeal, oat bran, nuts, seeds, legumes, beans, dried peas, lentils, apples, pears, strawberries, and blue berries. Insoluble fibers, which have a laxative effect, include whole wheat bread, barley, brown rice, whole grain cereals, and wheat bran.

Tips to increase your fiber intake:

-Eat whole fruits instead of fruit juice.

-Replace white rice, bread, and pasta with brown rice and whole grain products.

-Whole grain cereals.

-Snack on raw vegetables instead of chips or chocolate bars.

BCAA- Branch Chain Amino Acids are made up of 3 essential amino acids that cannot be produced by your body. BCAA's make up one third of skeletal muscle.

Taking BCAA supplements will help prevent muscle loss and will encourage visceral fat loss. Visceral fat is fat that accumulates around your organs and your abdominal area. You can maximize fat loss and retain your muscle mass because BCAA's are rapidly absorbed into the blood stream.

Probiotics- Probiotics are very important for assimilation of nutrients through the digestive tract and help to maintain good bacteria.

The Time Is Now

It is easy to plan out your day and then suddenly decide that those plans can wait till tomorrow, or the next day. I live by the old saying "don't do something tomorrow that you can do today!"

When I fought professionally in martial arts I had a goal and that goal was to win! If I walked out of that ring not victorious I knew that at the very least I gave 100%, and that just fueled my desire to train harder in preparing myself for my next match!

It takes discipline to strength train regularly. It is easy to procrastinate and the hardest part of any workout is thinking about starting. You just need to do it. These same principles can be applied to life itself. Apply this mind set to your GS20 Body Blast routines and you will be very well rewarded!

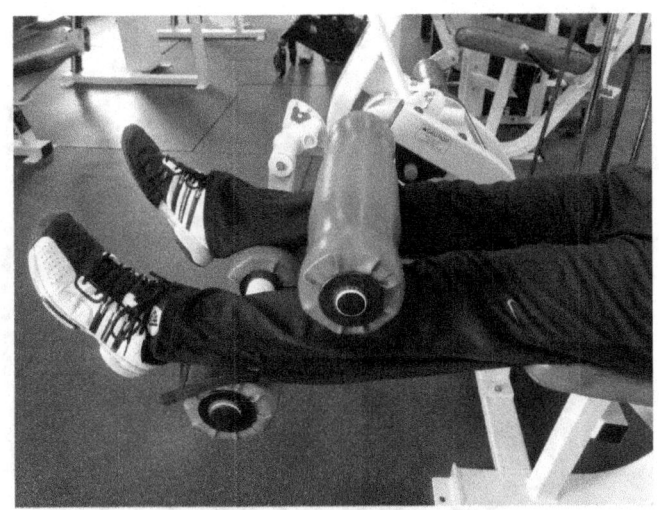

Leg Curl and Leg Extension: Proper seat positioning will ensure your knee lines up with the axis of rotation (as represented by the red knob on the side of the right knee)

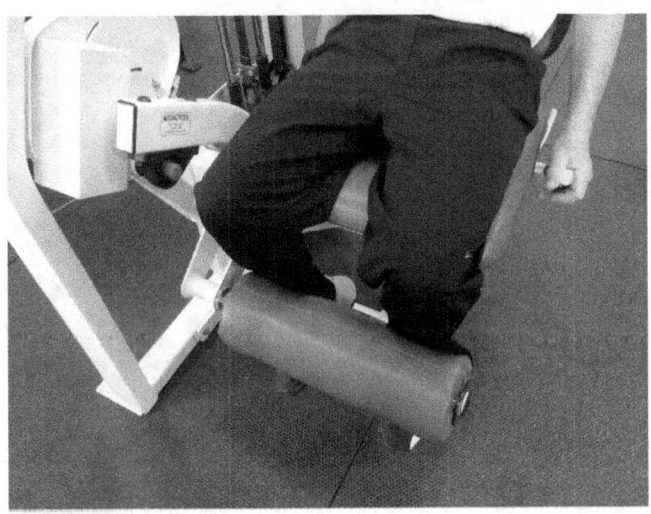

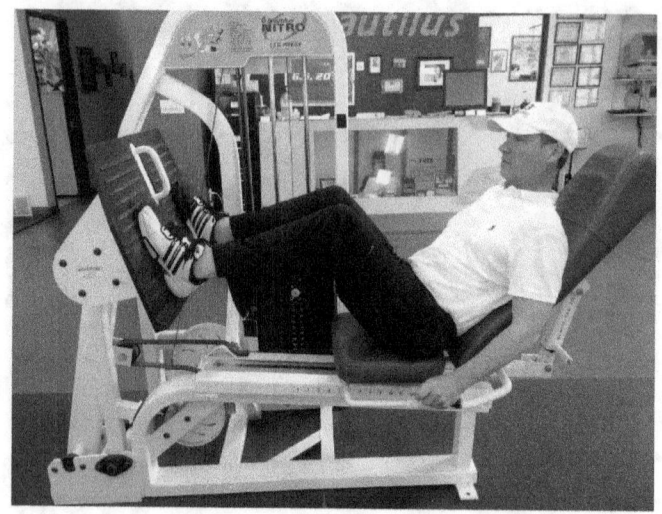

The Leg Press can be one of the most grueling exercises you do in the gym, but it had to be performed correctly. Be sure to not lock your legs out as this will transfer the weight load to the skeletal system and defeat the purpose of the exercise. Also be sure to exhale on the positive motions and inhale on the negative mostions

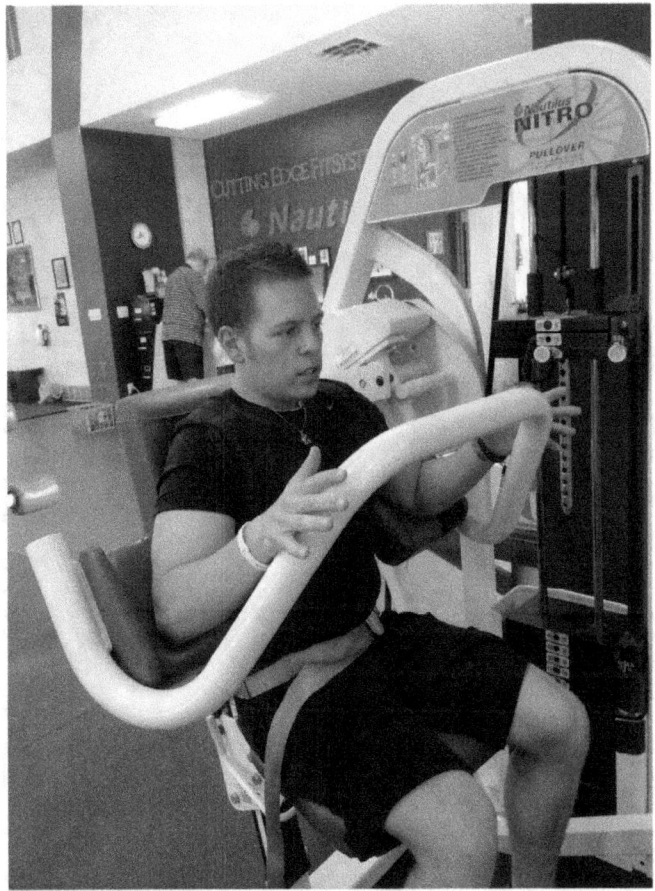

Pullover: Proper form on the pullover machine includes keeping and open hand on the bar. Griping the bar causes you to engage more of your arms during the exercise rather than your lat's, which is the muscle group you're focusing on.

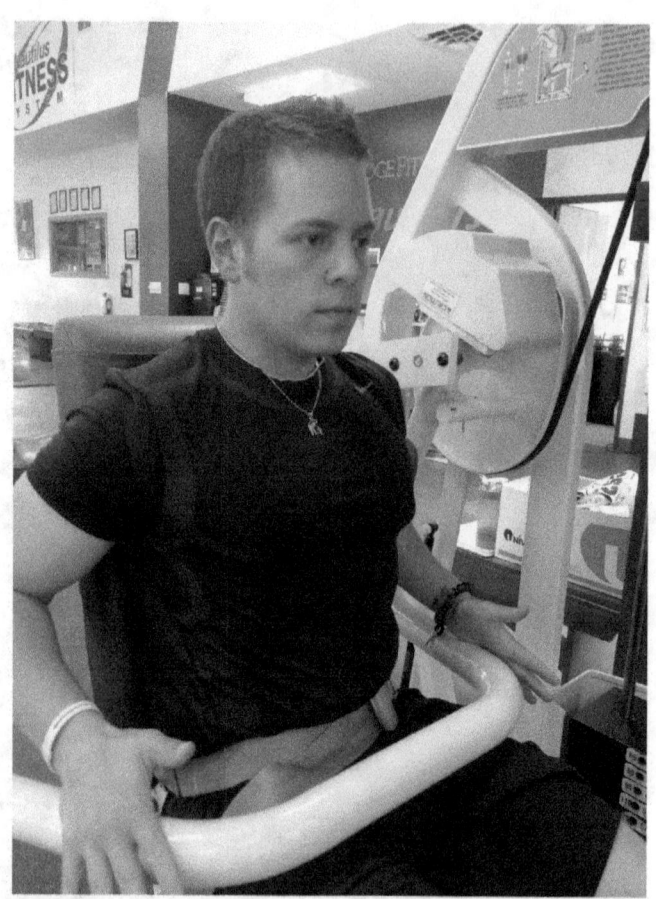

Pullover: Proper seat heigth ensures that your shoulders ae lined up with the axis of rotation. This allows the entire weight load to be lifted by the intended muscle group.

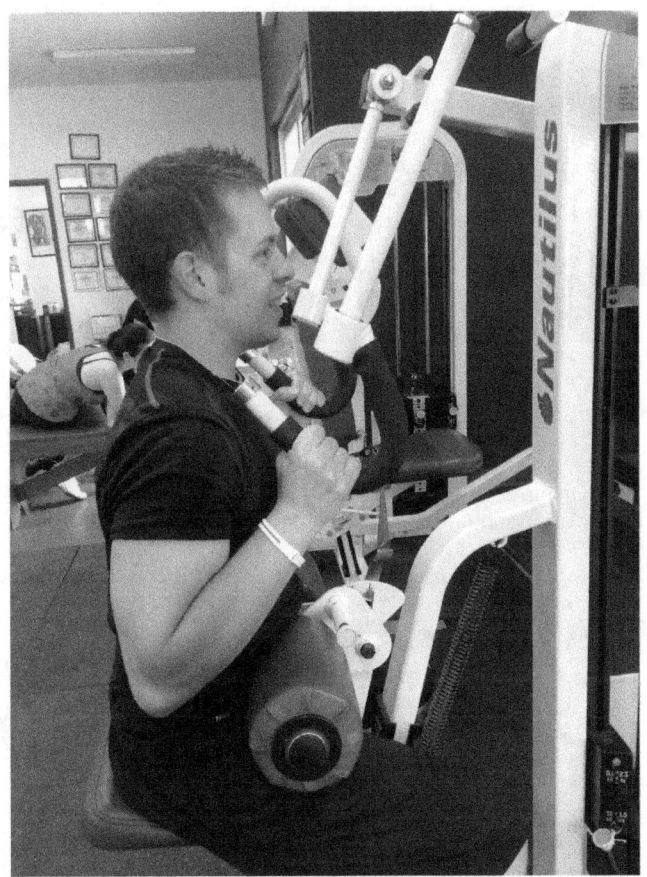

Lat. Pulldown: Regardless of the palm position, when performing Lat. Pulldown be sure to fully contract the muscles by bringing the handles down to your chest and holding that postition for one full second.

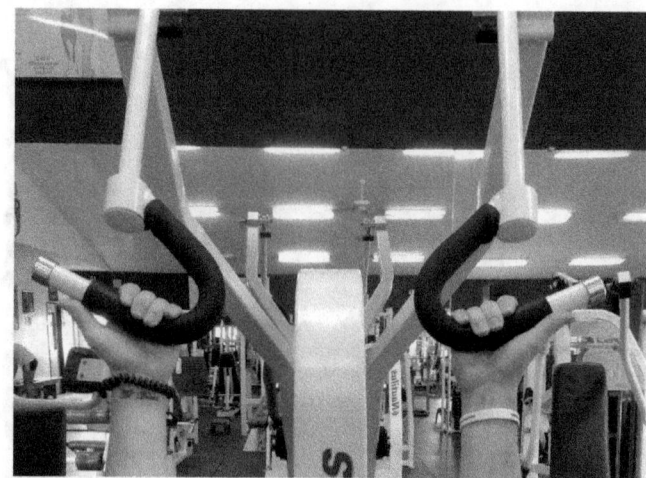

Top: Displays the palm-up style grip as utilized on the Lat. Pulldown machine.

Bottom: Displays the palm-in style grip as utilized on the Lat. Pulldown machine.

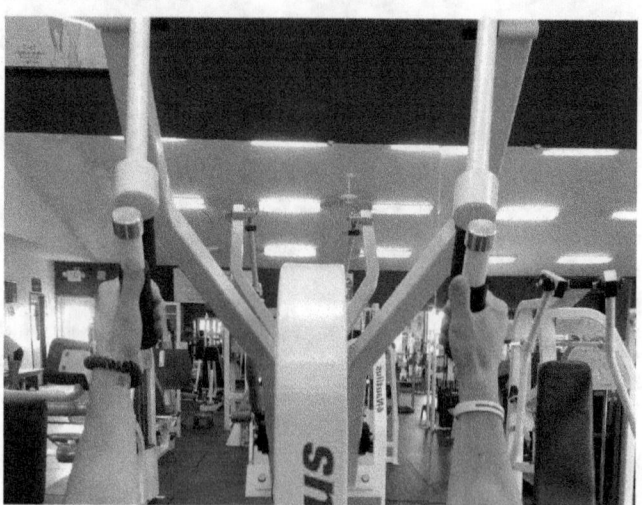

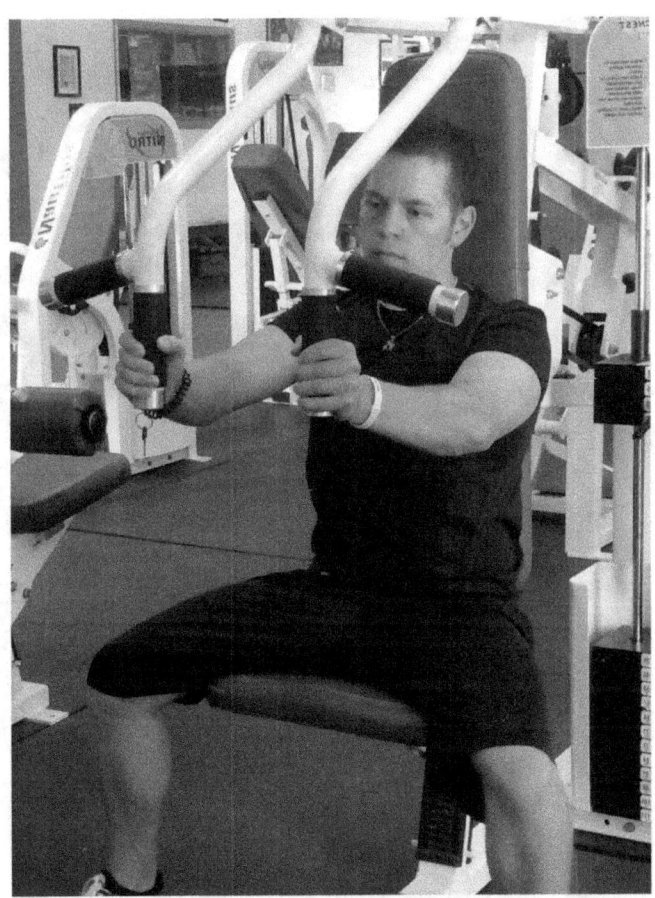

Vertical Chest (V-Chest): During pushing exercises remember to not lock-out your joints. This transfers the weight-load from the intended muscle group to the skeletal structure and can cause damaged with long-term effects.

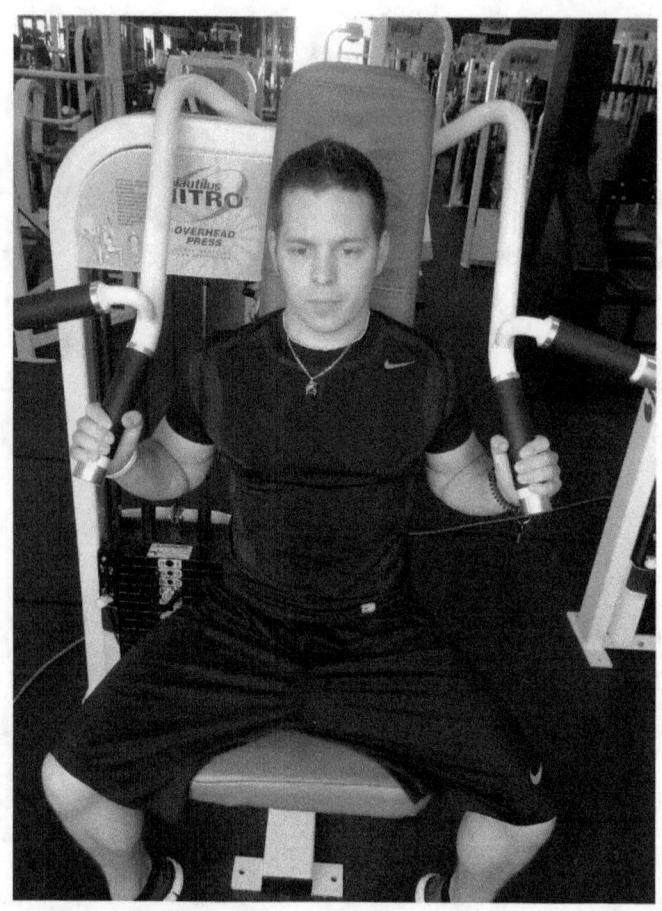

Overhead Press: A proper seat postion will bring your shoulders to be lined up with the horizontal grip handles.

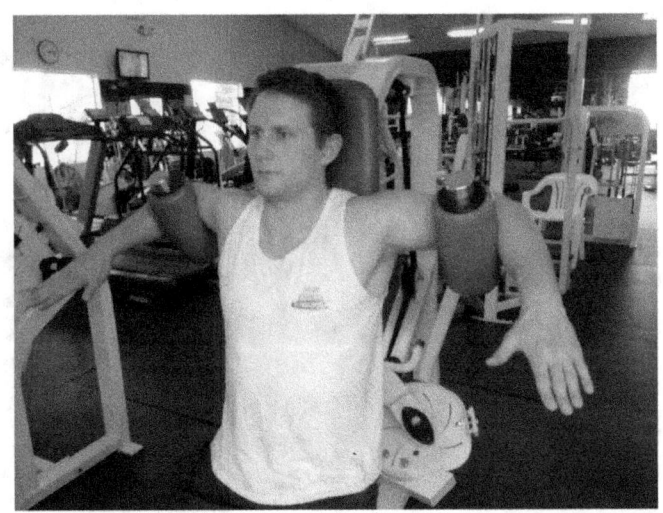

Starting and ending positions on the Nautilus Pec Fly machine.

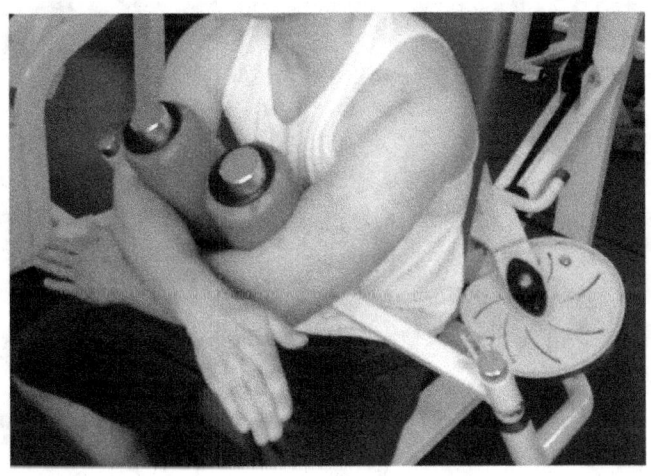

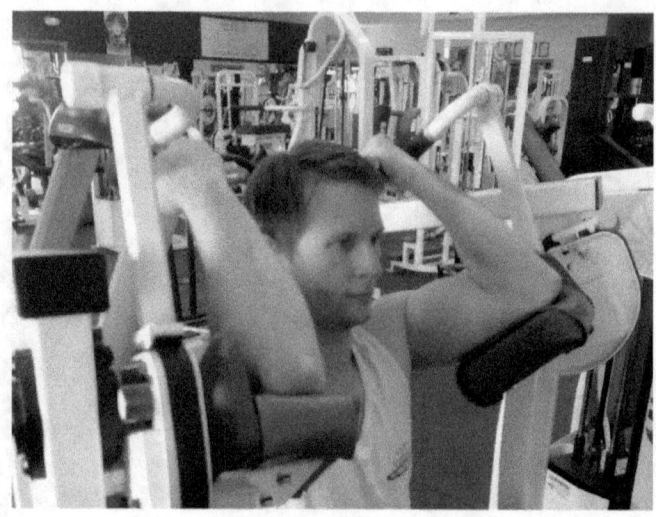

The Bicep and Tricep machines have an axis of rotation that lines up with the center of your elbow.

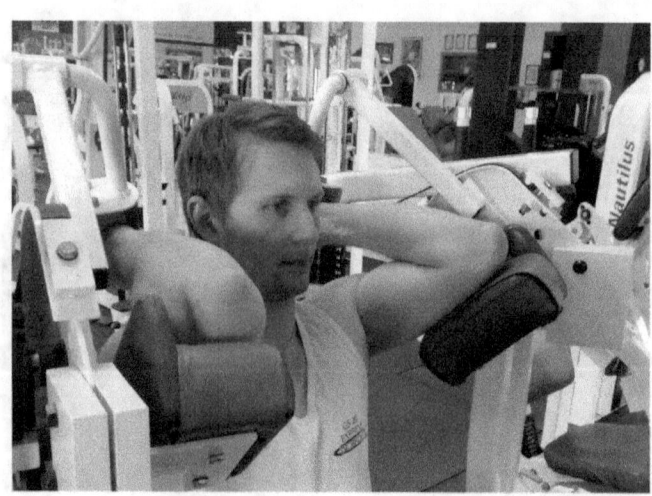

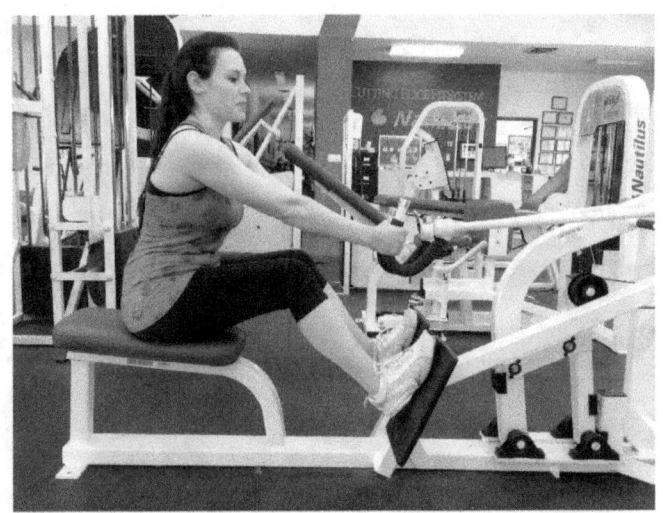

Starting and finishing positions for the row machine.

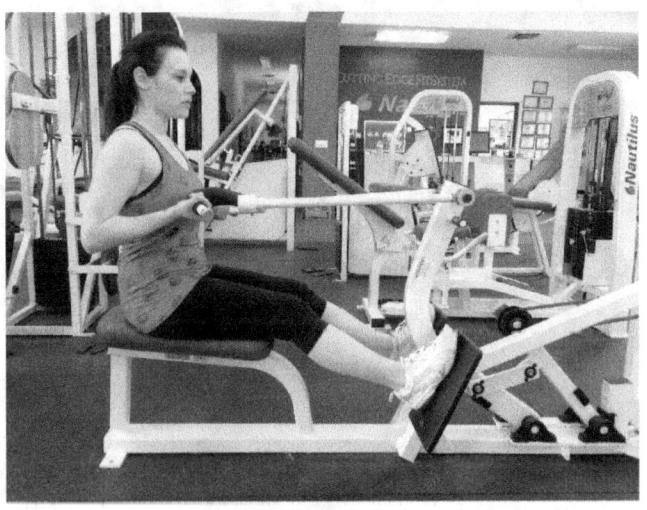

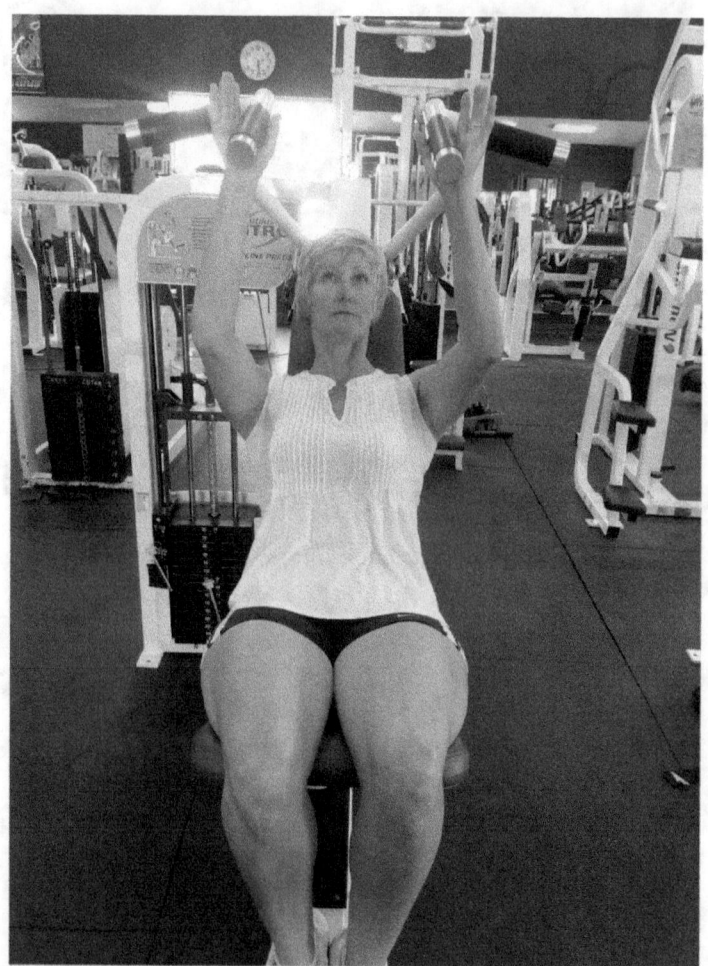

On the incline press machine, as with all pushing movements, be sure to keep a loose and open grip while making sure to not lock outthe joint being used (in this case your elbows)

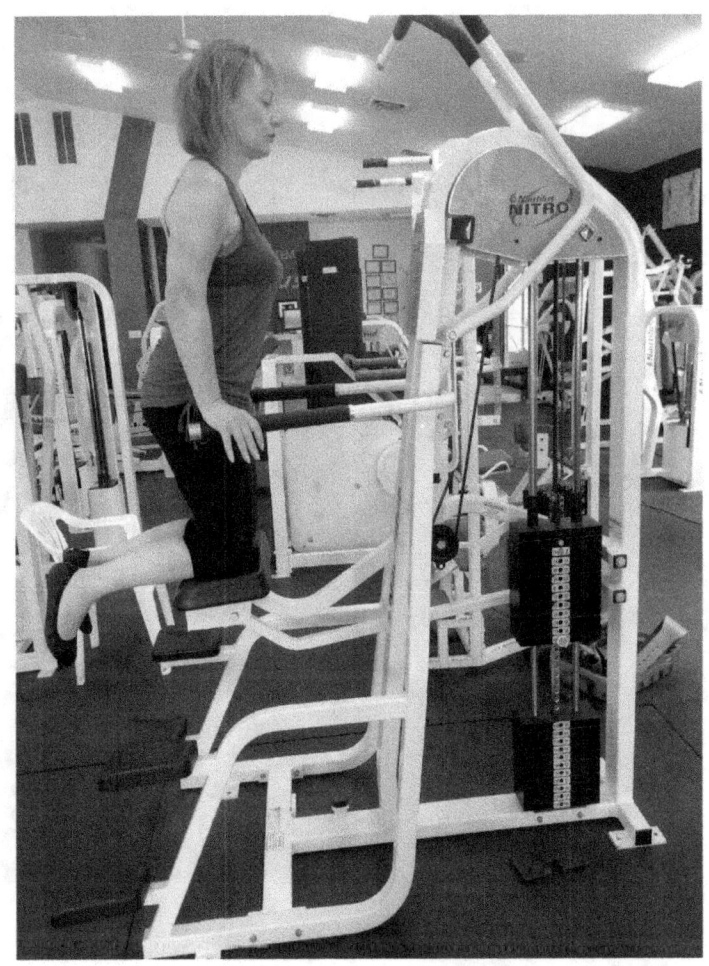

Performing assisted dips on the gravitron machine.

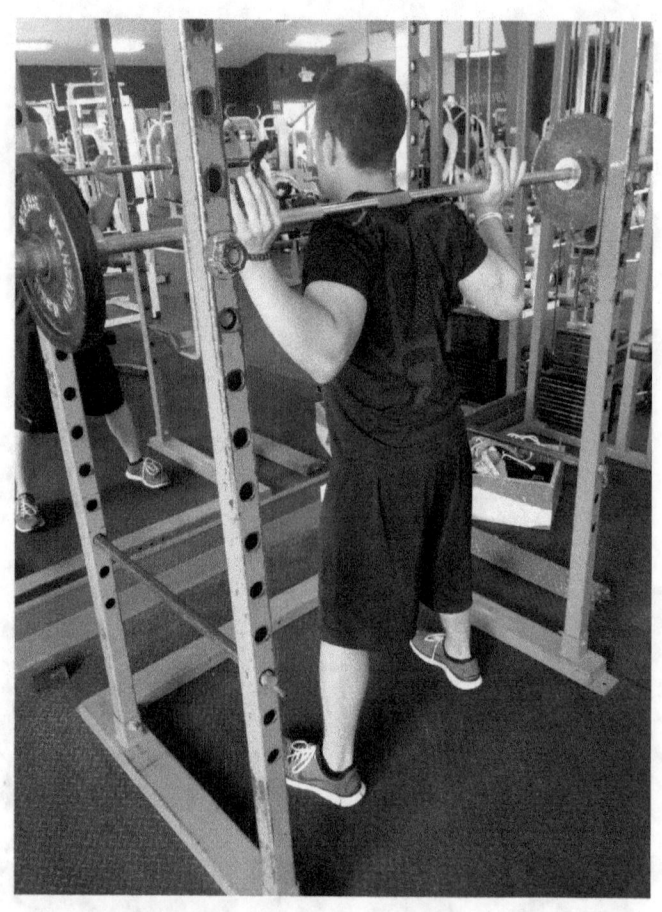

Starting position for the barbell squat.

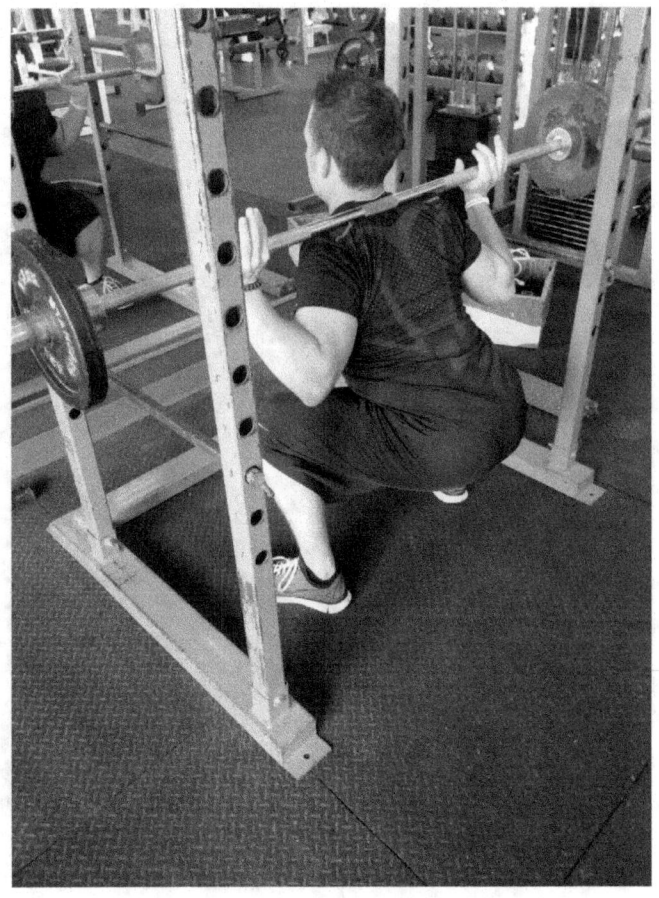

Finishing position for the barbell squat.

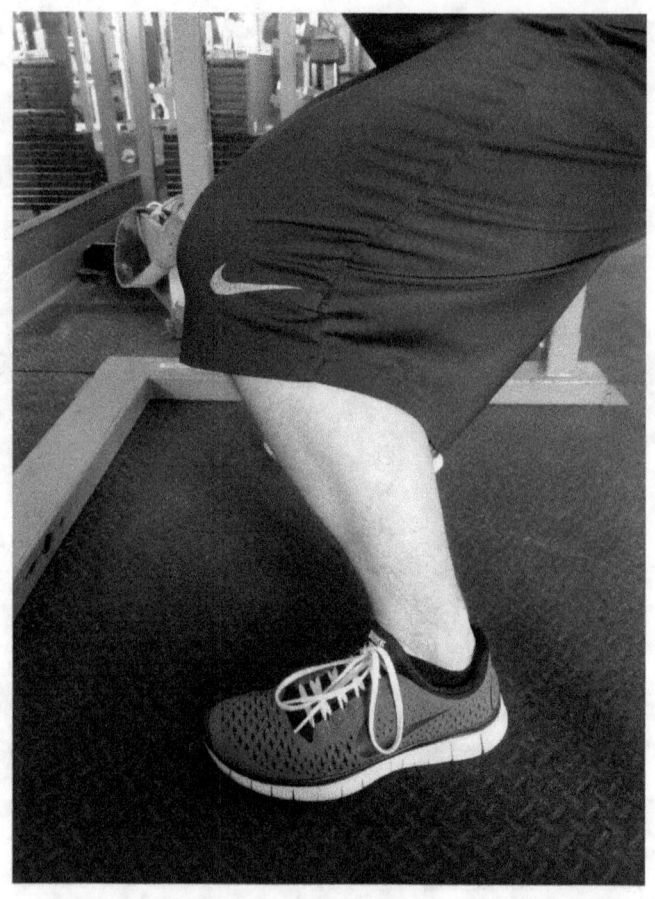

Maintaining a proper stance and footing during the barbell squat is just as critical to safety as it is to getting the most out of the exercise.

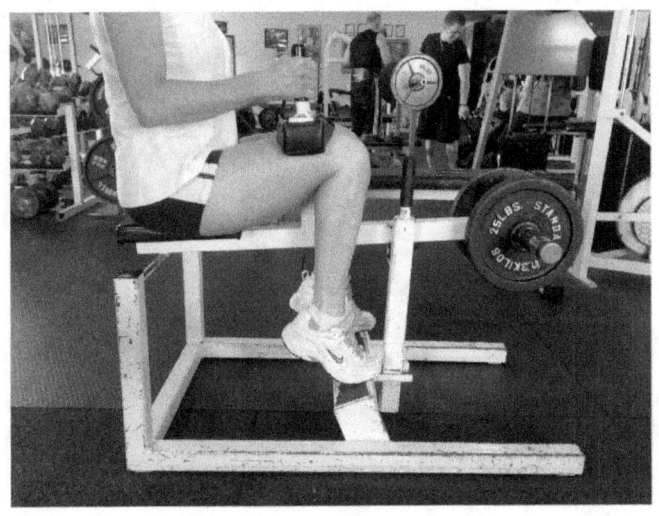

The seated calf-raise is one of the best ways to isolate and
fully-exhaust your calf muscles.

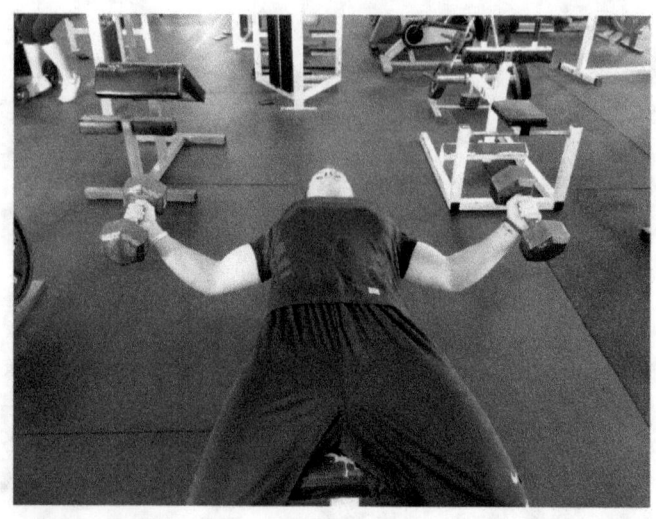

Starting and finishing positions for the flat bench dumbbell flys.

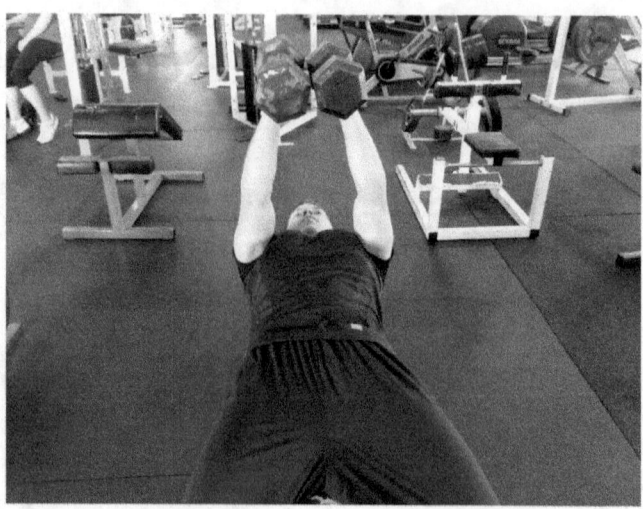

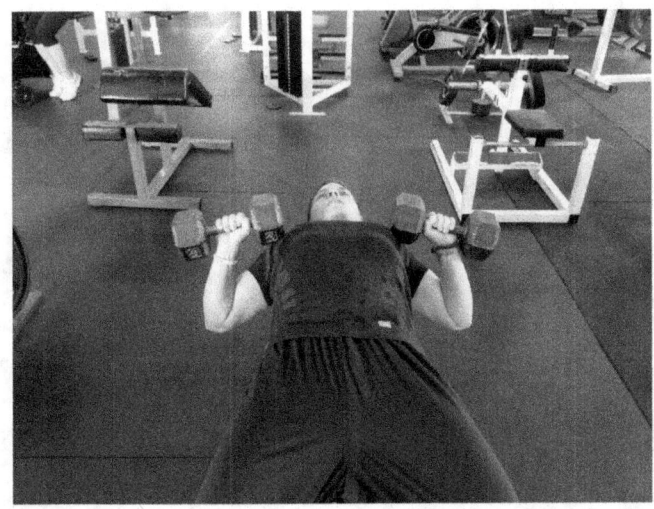

Starting and finishing positions for the flat bench dumbbell press.

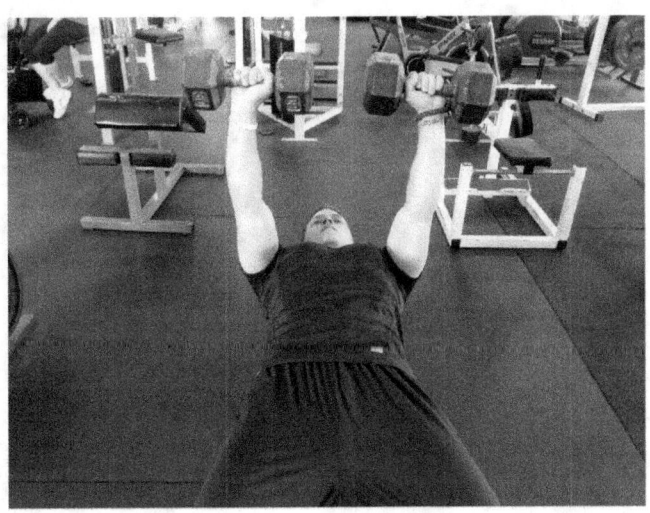

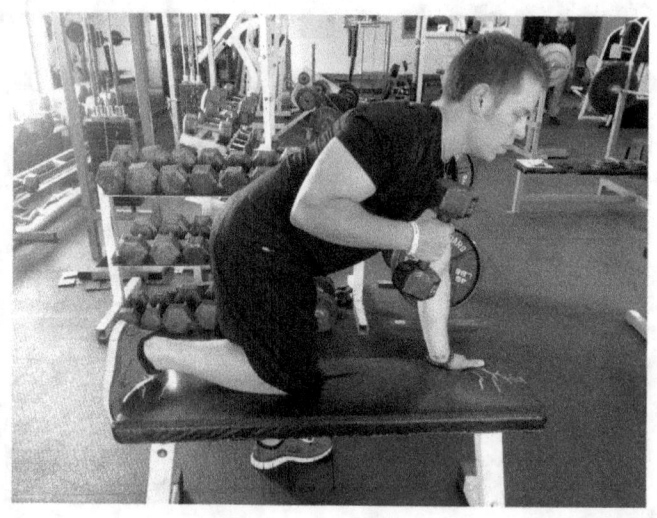

Starting and finishing positions for the tricep kickbacks with dumbbells.

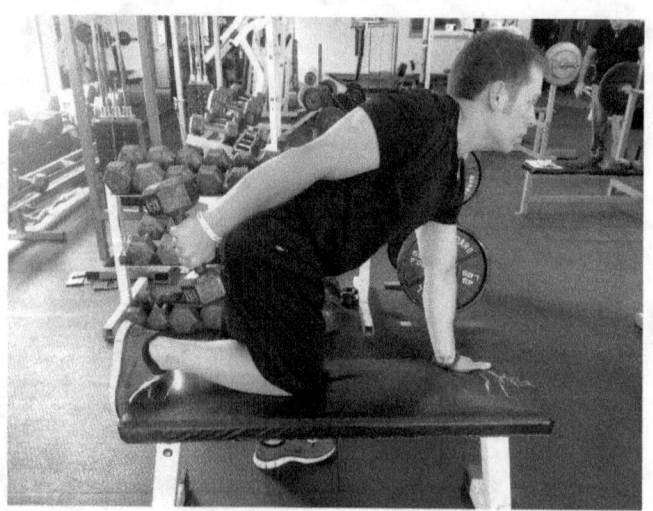

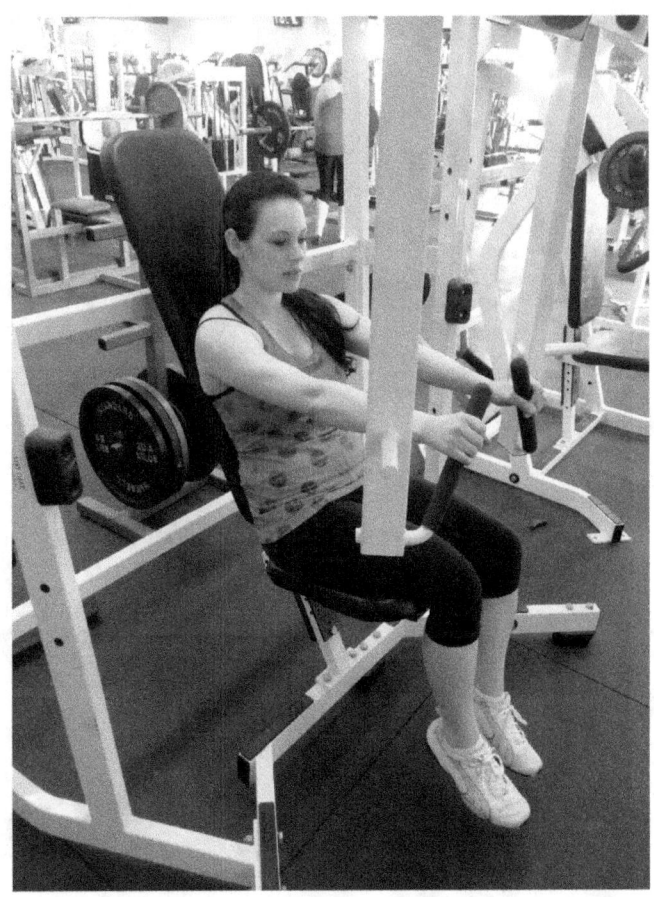

Plate loaded machines (such as this plate loaded vertical chest machine) can work just as well as selectorized equipment if you have no selectorized options.

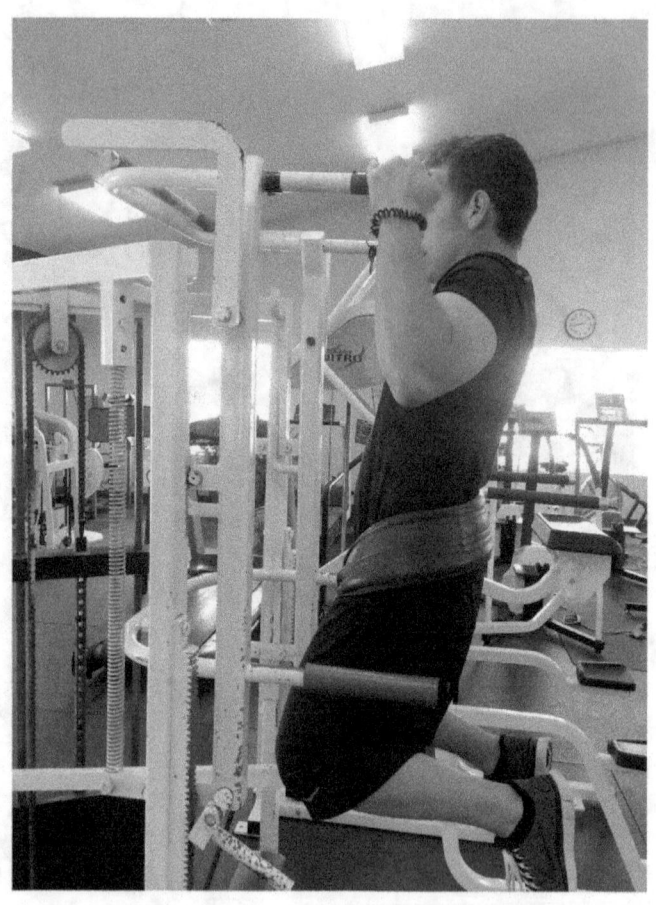

Starting position for negative chins (wide grip).

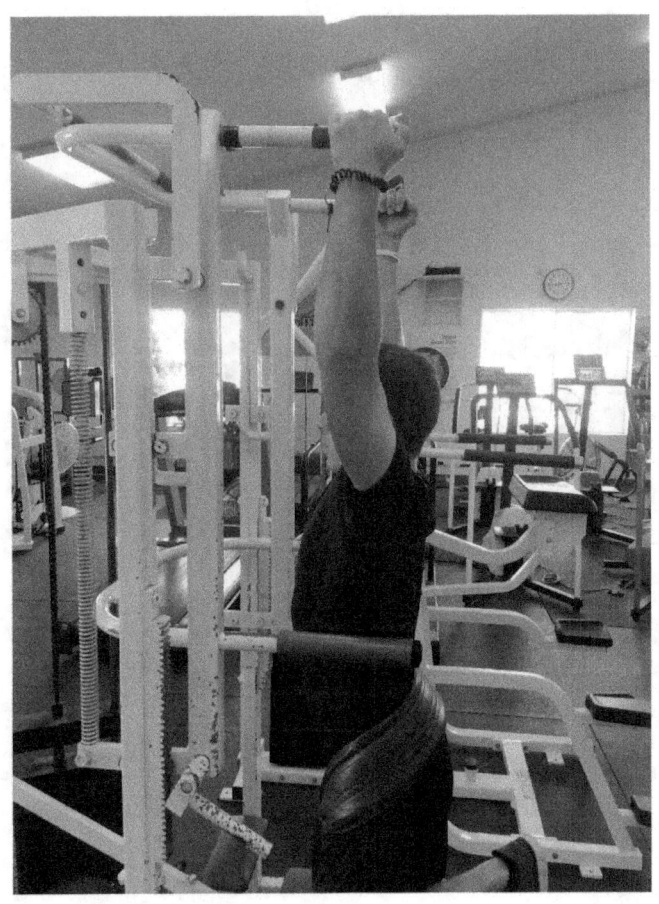

Finishing position for negative chins (wide grip).

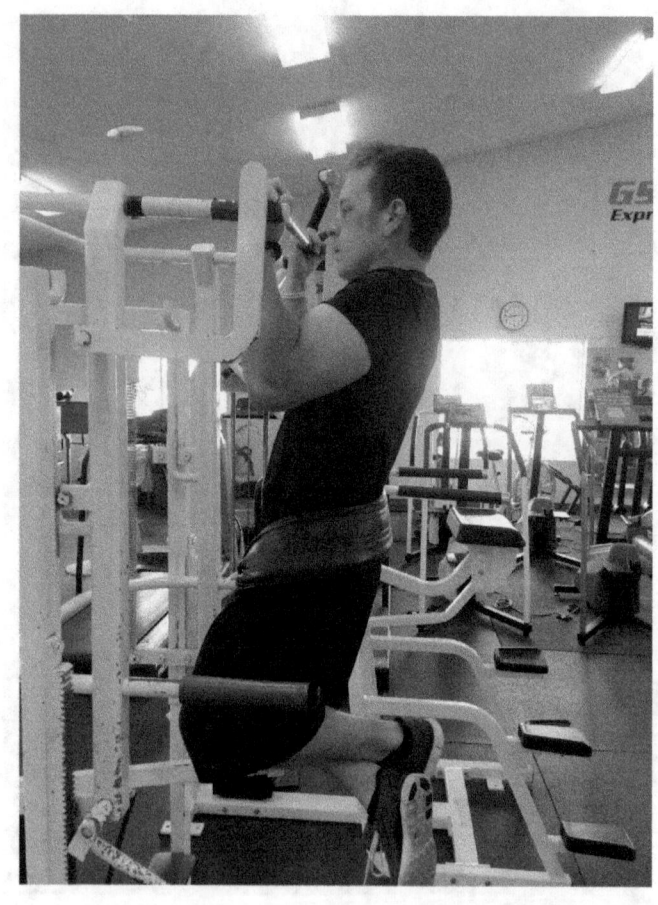

Starting position for negative chins (regular grip).

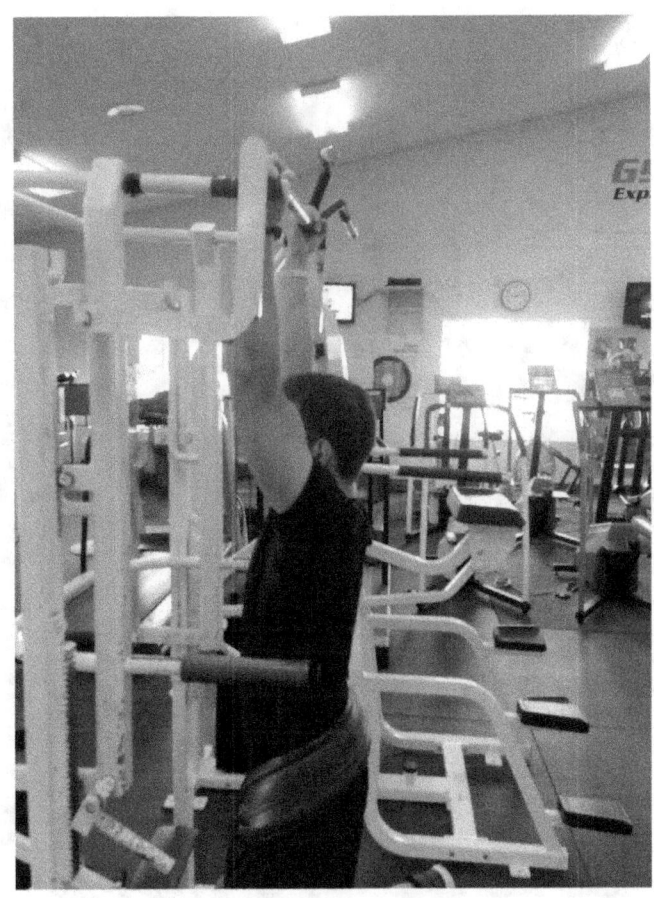

Finishing position for negative chins (regular grip).

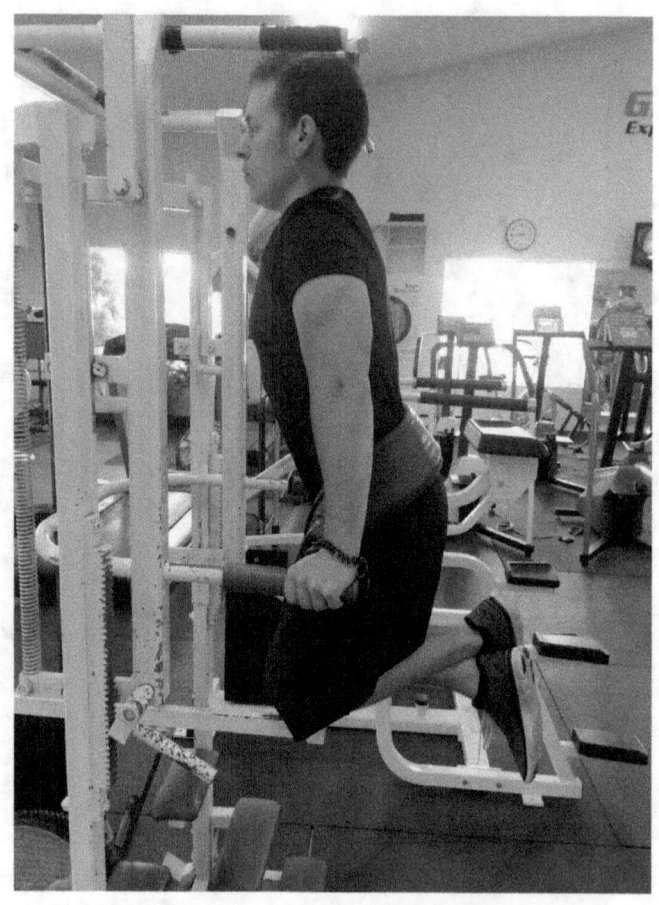

Starting position for negative dips (regular grip).

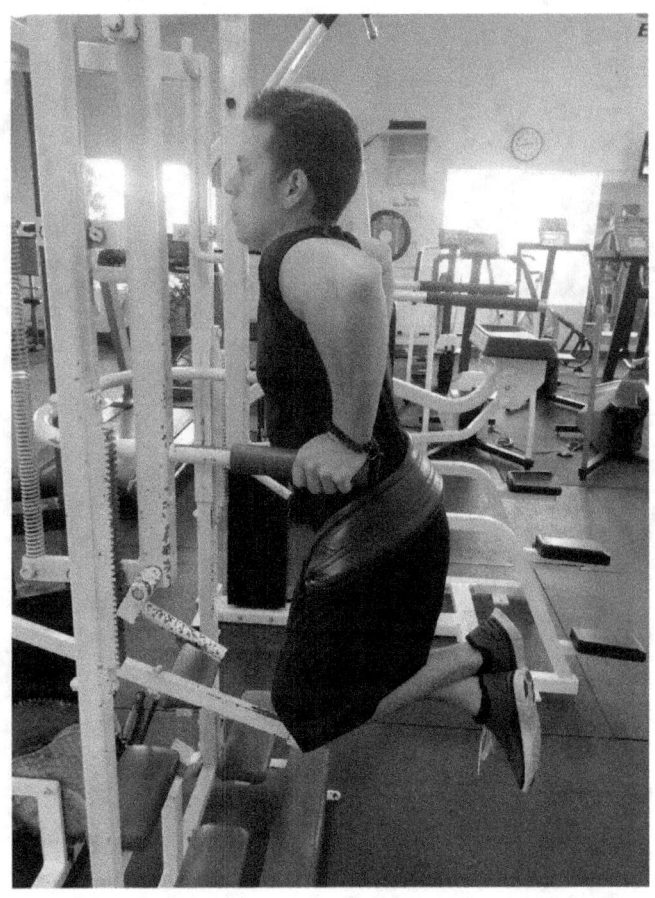

Finishing position for negative dips (regular grip).

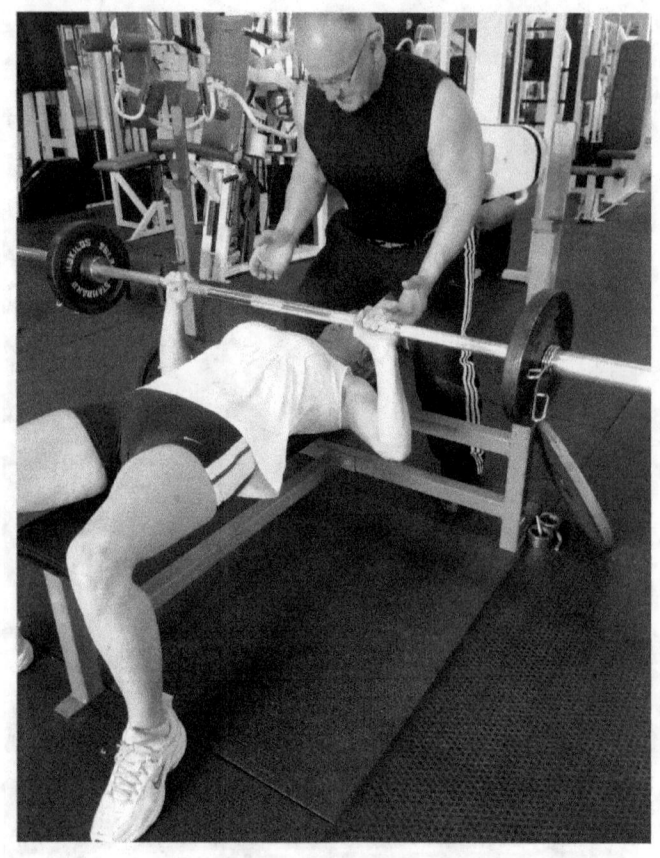

Starting positions for the flat bench barbell press. Remember that using a spotter can help you maximize results when performing free-weight exercises.

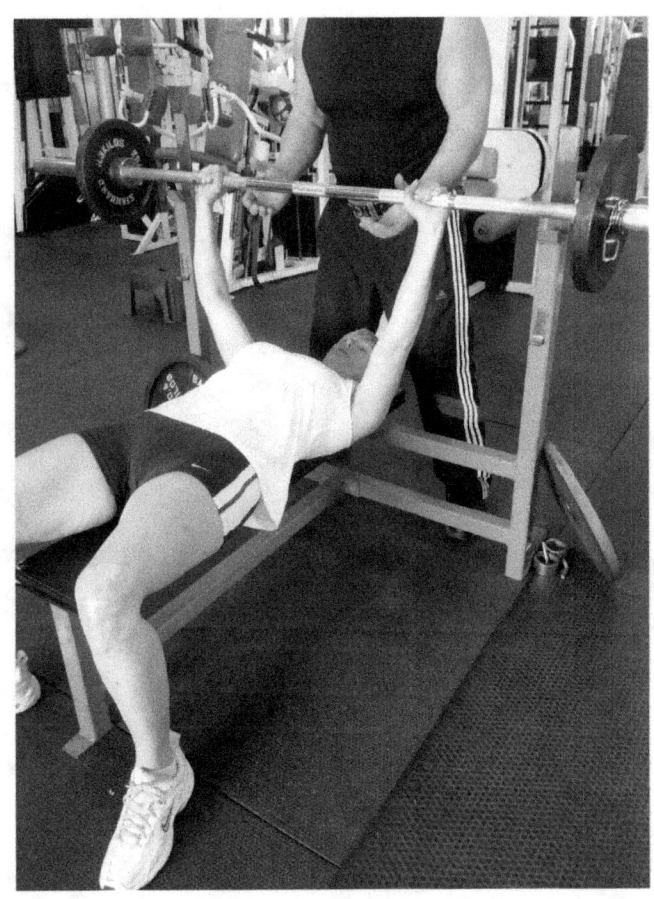

Finishing position for the flat bench barbell press.

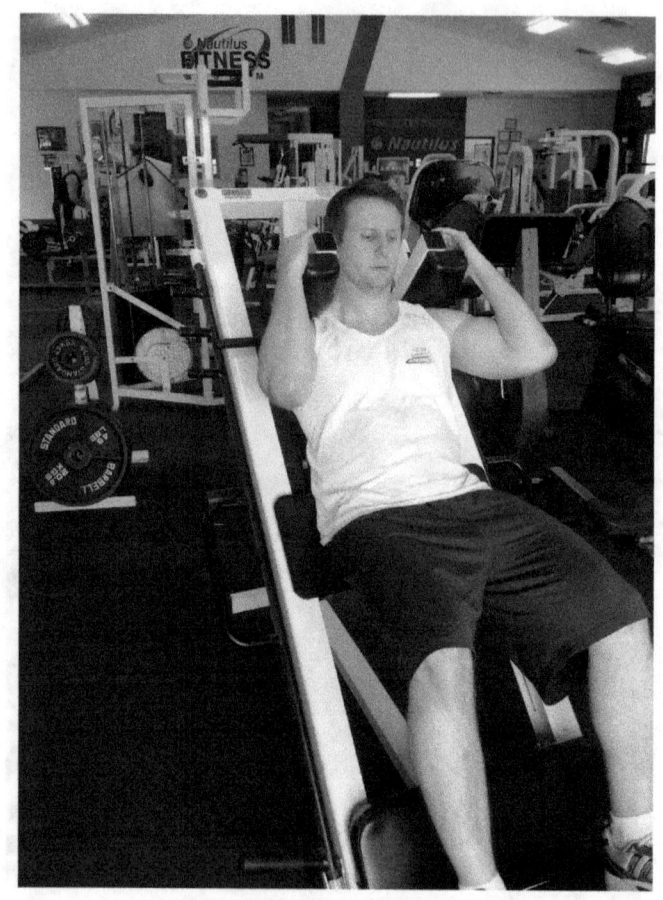

Hack squat using the hip sled

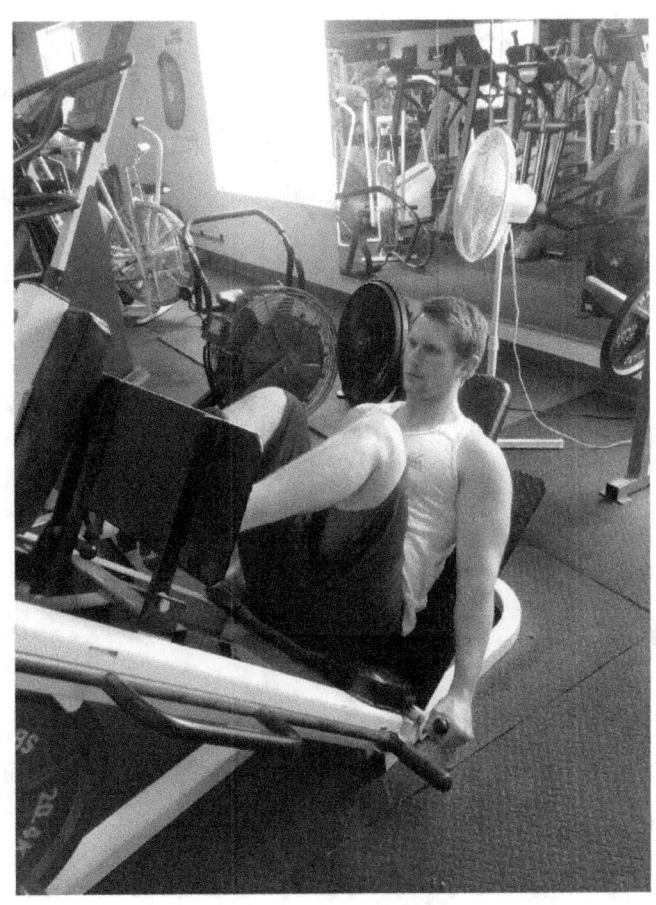

Leg press using the hip sled

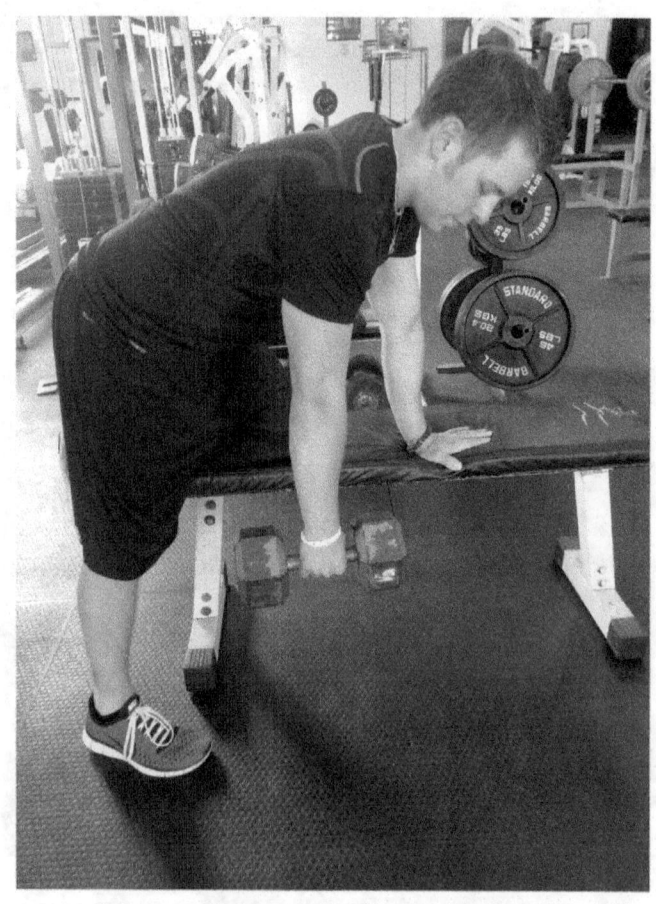

One-arm bent-over row starting position.

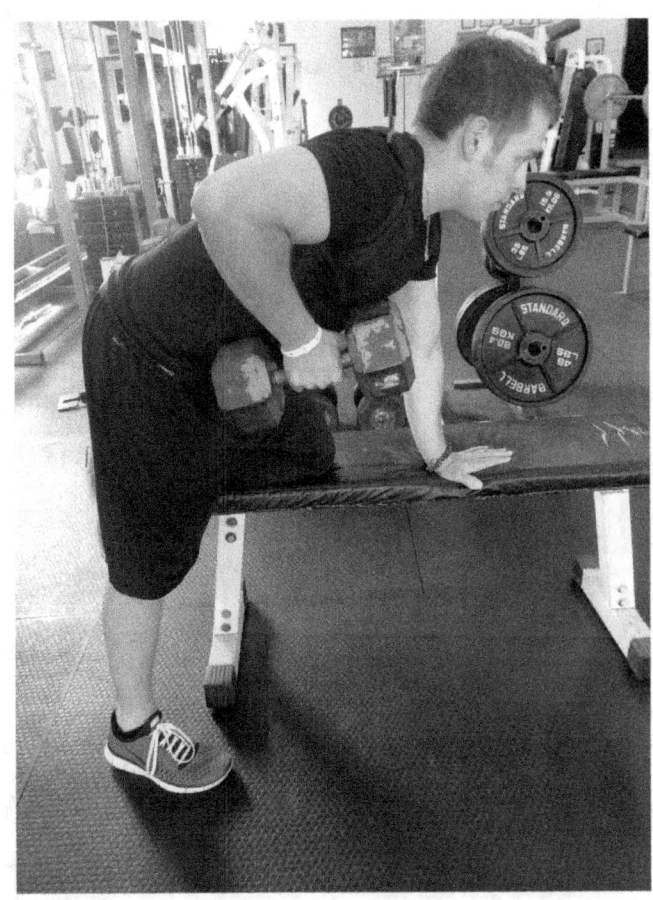

One-arm bent-over row finishing position.

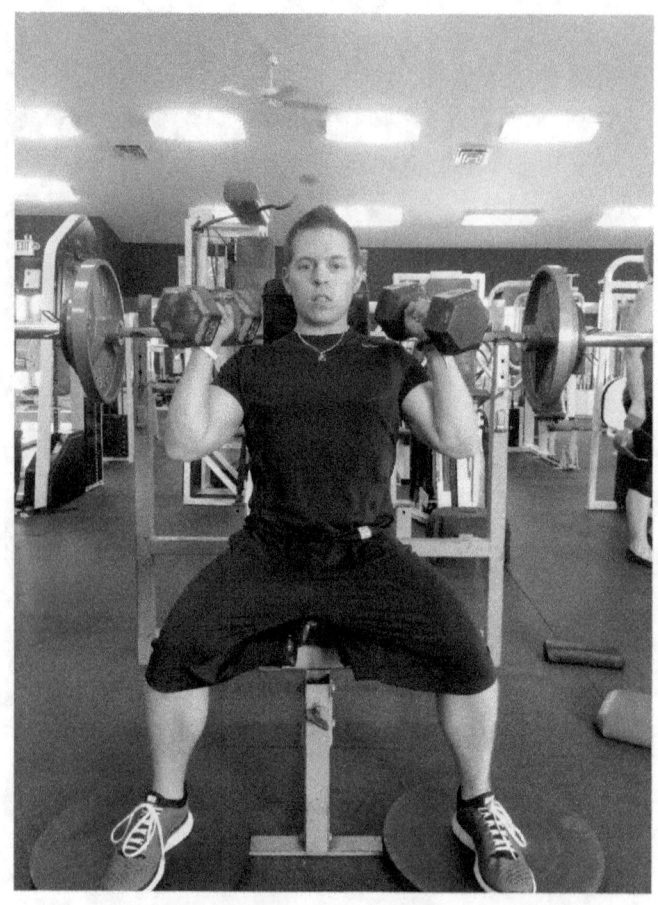

Seated dumbbell press starting position.

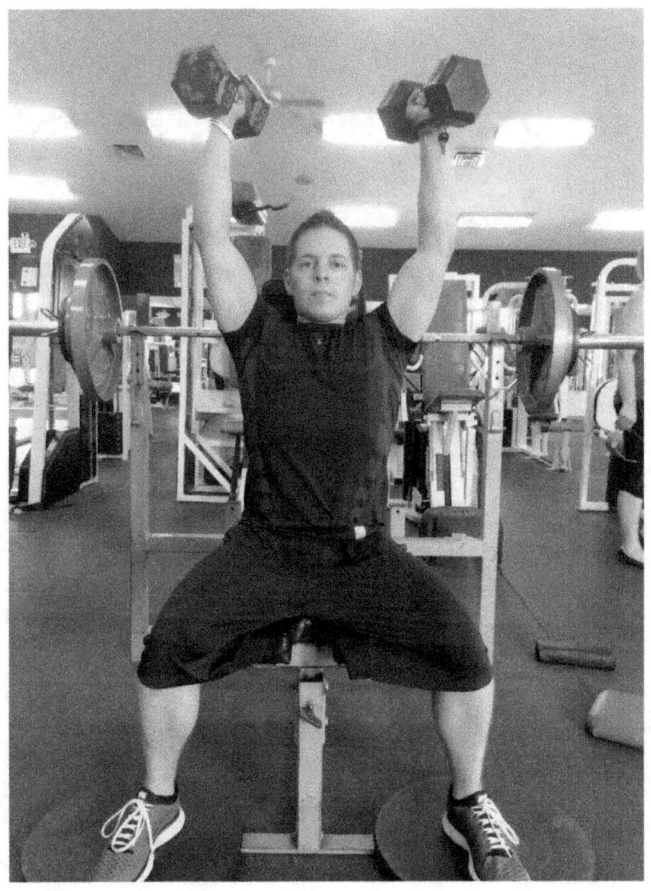

Seated dumbbell press finishing position.

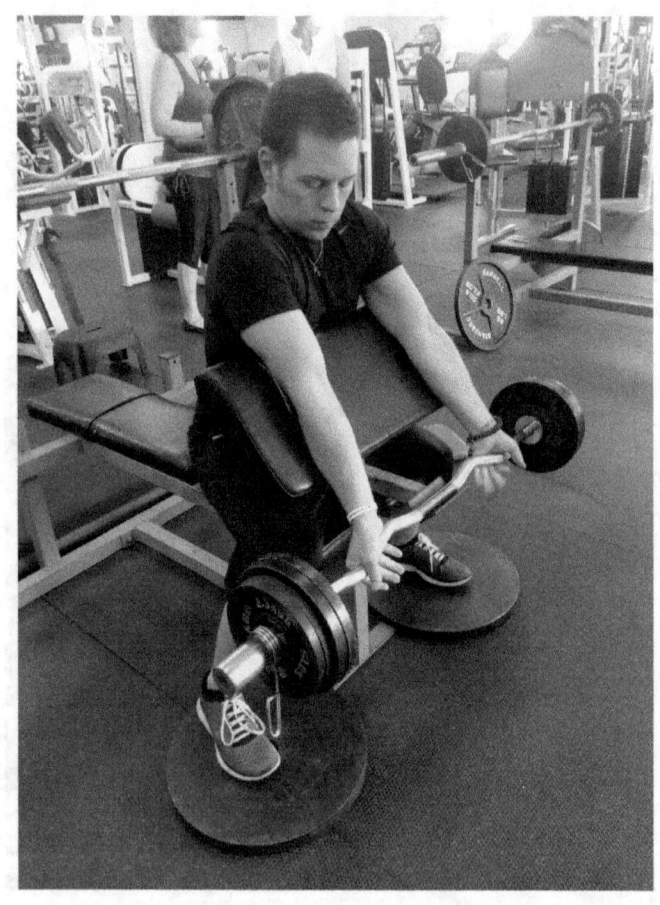

Preacher curl starting position.

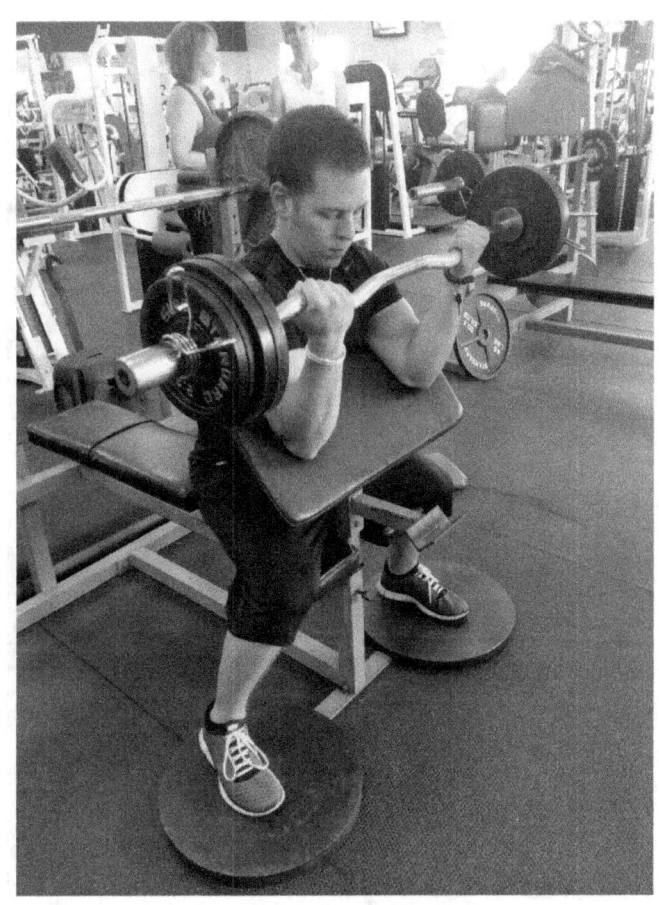

Preacher curl finished position.

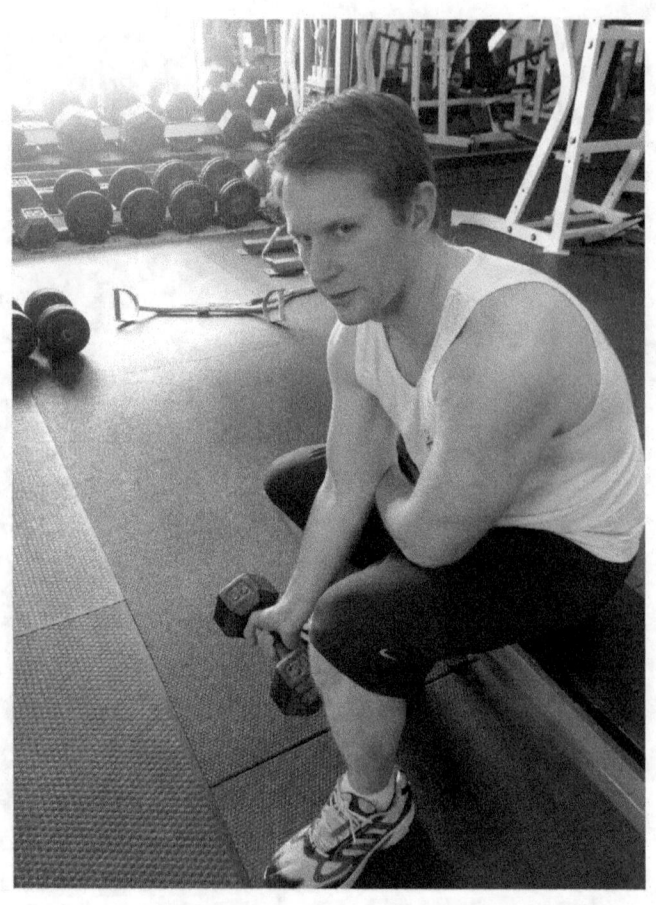

Isolated bicep curl starting position.

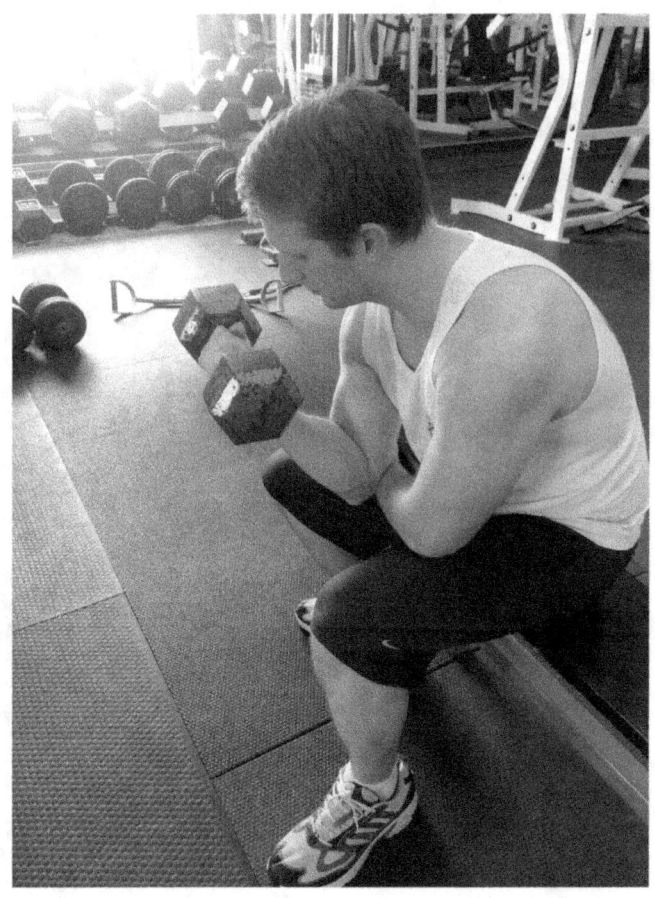

Isolated bicep curl finished position.

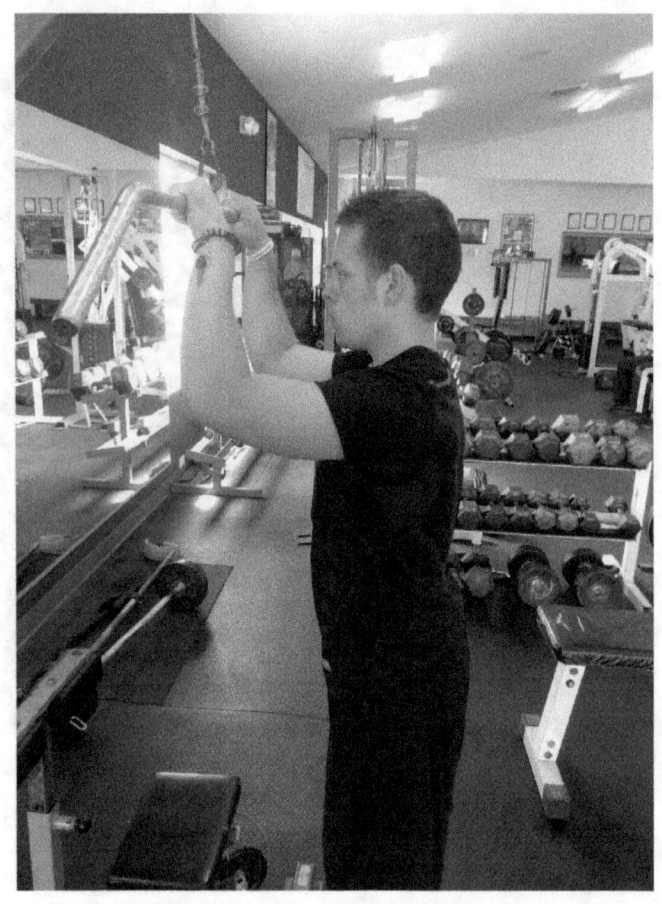

Tricep push downs starting position.

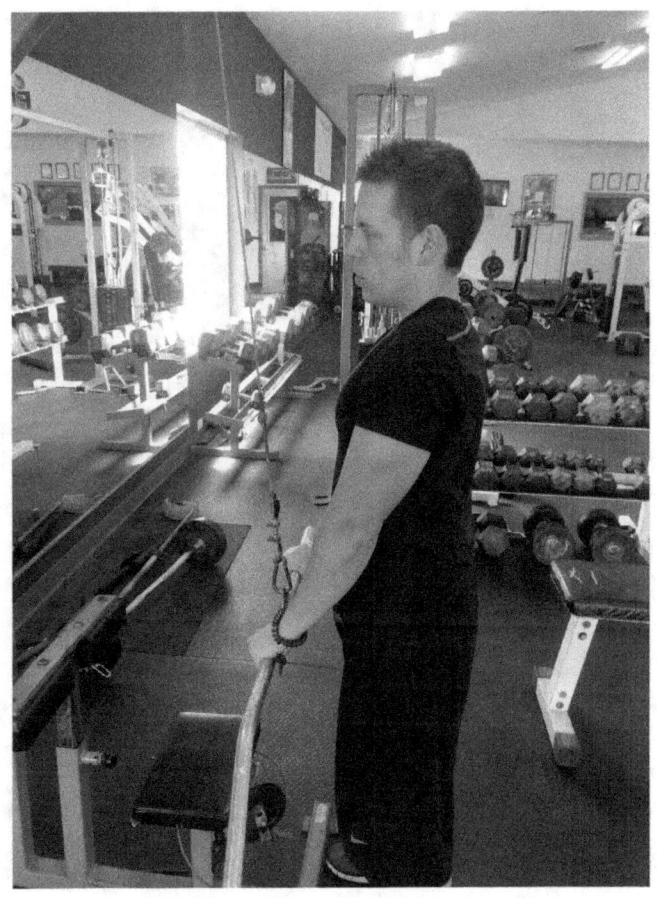

Tricep push downs finished position.

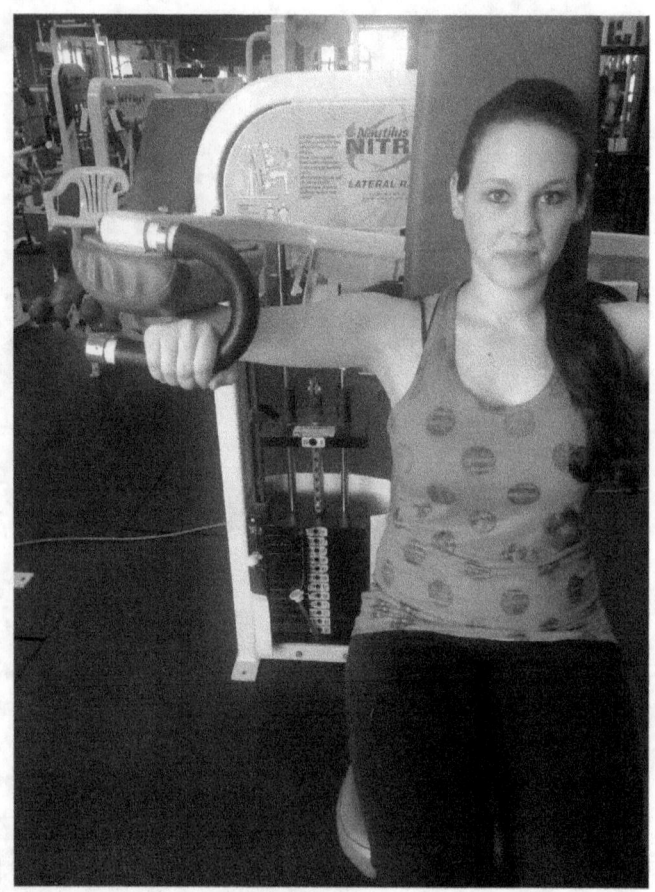

When performing the lateral raise your arms should stop when they are parallel with the ground. Many people make the mistake of raising their arms higher than this which increases the risk of injury and expells unnecessary energy.

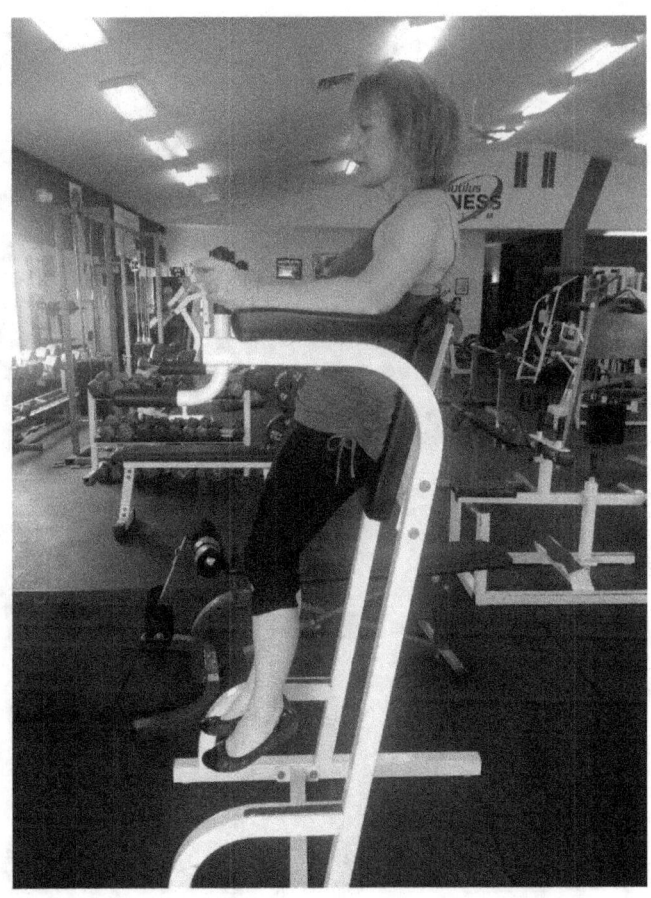

Leg raises starting position.

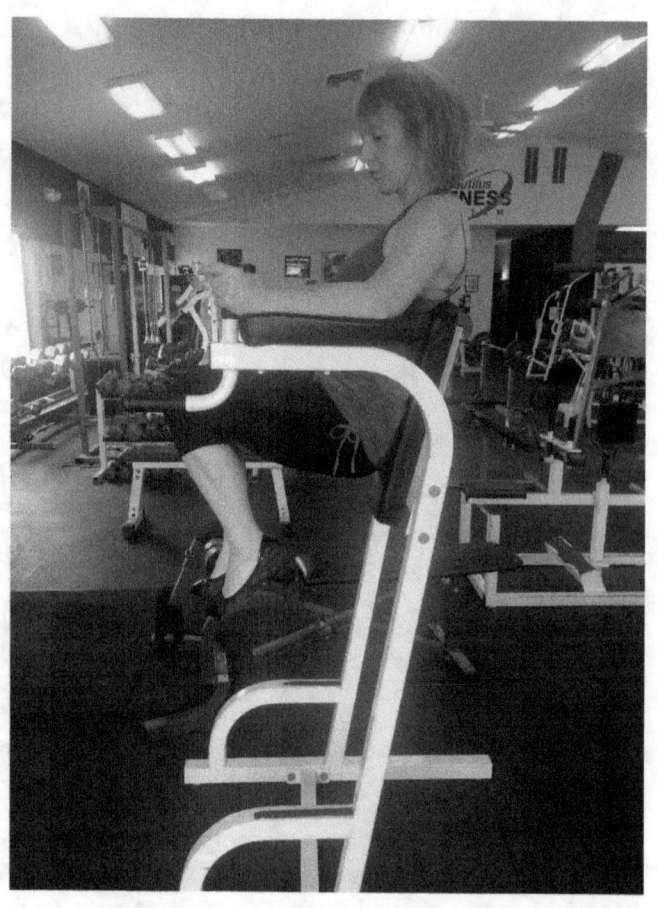

Leg raises finished position.

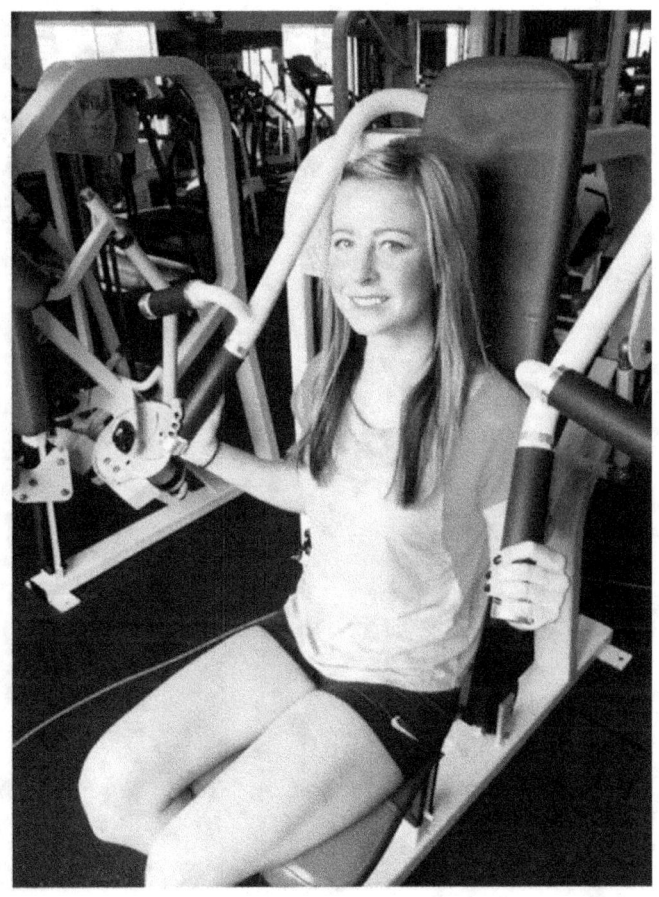

Proper seating height on the overhead press.

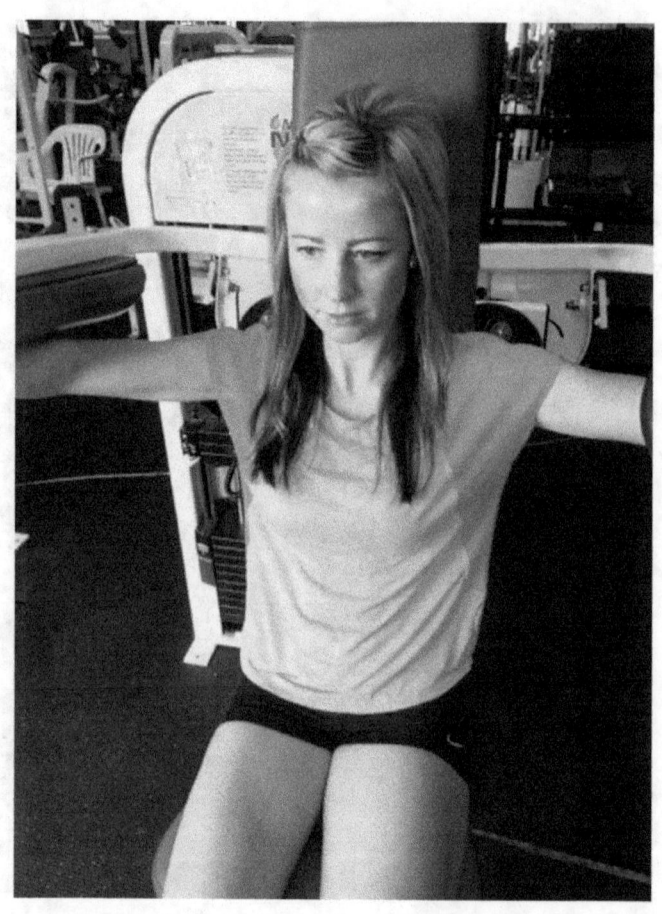

Proper rep range on the lateral raise.

TESTIMONIALS

With my professional career as a physician, the GS20 workout has been a perfect fit for me. It provides a structured, efficient, exercise routine that blends well with a busy work schedule. The equipment and exercises used, make it a safe and controlled environment, not putting one at a high risk of injury. I believe anyone who commits to the GS20 will find very rewarding benefits in health and strength!

Michael Harbryl, D.O.
Ophthalmologist

I have a clinic at Gary's exercise facility, and I have been using the GS20 exercise program for almost 20 years. I think it's a great exercise plan that works the entire body in 20 minutes. The plan changes every eight weeks; the muscle, ligament, and tendon systems are stimulated by doing the new formats of exercise. This maximizes the health benefits to those systems and circulation, nerve stimulation, the bone system, etc. It's an exercise plan that can be utilized by both men and women. I recommend it for better health.

Ronald J. Looney, D.C.
Chiropractor

The GS20 has been a game changer for me. The program has provided a structured, challenging but achievable means to exercise health. I have recommended the program to several of my patients of all ages and abilities, with rewarding results.

Louis S. Habryl, D.O. FAOAO
Orthopedic Surgeon

I have trained under Gary for 30+ years using the concepts of his GS20 style of training. Staying in shape gave me confidence mentally and physically while performing the taxing duties of police work.

At a recent physical exam, my doctor told me that at age 70, my level of fitness was in the top 5% of all age groups 40 years and up! I attribute this to Gary and the GS20 program.

Walt Mikula
Retired Lieutenant
Michigan Conservation Officer
40 years in Law Enforcement

I am a 56 year-old female who began the GS20 workout six months ago. Three months into the program, I began to tell my husband on a daily basis, "I feel so GOOD!" I would repeat this several times a day! I felt strong, toned, less stressed, and my sleep patterns improved. I think my husband was tired of hearing it because the next thing I knew he joined the gym and started the GS20 program.

I am a registered nurse with an ANCC certification in psychiatric and mental health nursing. The GSO20 workout is part of my personal wellness plan. Thanks Gary!

Debbie McCann, RN-BC

As a registered nurse I have to stay strong physically to do my job, which often involves lifting patients. As the primary caregiver for my elderly parents, time (or lack thereof) is a big factor in my life. The GS20 workout fits in perfectly with my busy life. I have increased my strength and flexibility dramatically.

Charlene Goszczynski, RN

As a busy wife, mom, and nurse, I always felt that I didn't have time to work out. The GS20 workout changed that for me. It's fast, yet delivers results. Anyone can find time to do it! I'm in the best shape I have ever been. The GS20 workout changed my life!

Rene Ames, RN BSN

The GS20 program has made it possible for me to workout consistently for the past 10 years. Through college, careers, children, and daily life, I would have stopped working out years ago had I not been using a system that was fast, efficient, and proven effective. Most other exercise programs are not engaging enough to retain members long enough after they see some results, but the GS20 does. I know that with this program I will continue strength training for the rest of my life.

Stephan Kwapis

I have been exercising for 55 years, particularly strength training, and in the last 40 years we have learned a vast amount in the science of exercise. However, there remains a huge amount of misinformation and misunderstanding on the amount of exercise required to achieve the best possible results. Probably the main reason for this confusion is the various protocols out there claiming to have all the answers, we don't claim to have all the answers, but a lot more than most!

One thing I do know, "It takes very little exercise, properly performed to produce very good results", and I emphasize properly performed.

Even many world class bodybuilders make the mistake of overtraining. There is a wide variety of supplements they can take to create a false indication of being recovered from previous workouts. These supplements can make them feel stronger faster, but it is quite the contrary, ligaments, tendons, and the muscle structure itself are far from being recovered, and that is why on many occasions they experience torn muscles!

I reluctantly admit, that I have over-trained for 20 years and I knew better! Obviously, it is very easy to over-train.

In the last few years, I reduced the amount of exercise even more! That was the birth of my "Max Body Blast routines"

Even though I am now older, I am simply amazed at the results I never thought were possible.

"So when in doubt, do less" I will mention one more time, perform your repetitions very slow, when doing this you produce more "muscular force" - therefore greater muscle fiber recruitment (better results) and it is safe!

Follow the guidelines in my book, and it will lead you in the right direction.

Gary Stempien

JOIN THE GS20 FAMILY

Become a part of our Facebook pages to keep up to date on exercise secrets, correspond with fitness professionals, hear and share success stories, and much more!

www.facebook.com/gs20expressworkout
www.facebook.com/cuttingedgefitsystem

Visit our websites for additional fitness information and news. Plus, review a controlled study with one of our college athletes (the only way to find out the results is to visit us online)!

www.cuttingedgefitsystem.com
www.gs20expressworkout.com

www.ingramcontent.com/pod-product-compliance
Lightning Source LLC
Chambersburg PA
CBHW060355290526
45791CB00002B/517